# The Licensing Exam Review Guide in Nursing Home Administration

*Sixth Edition*

**James E. Allen, PhD, MSPH, CNHA**, is Associate Professor of Health Policy and Administration Emeritus at the University of North Carolina at Chapel Hill and President of LongTermCare Education.com, a national resource website for information on the long term care field. He has 30-plus years of experience teaching and conducting research in the field of health care administration. He taught courses at the University of North Carolina at Chapel Hill in long term care administration, medical ethics, and the organization and financing of health care delivery in the United States. He has provided legal consultation in long term care litigation matters across ten states.

The website www.longtermcareedu.com (or www.ltce.com) provides more than 500 pages of state-by-state, up-to-date information on such subjects as:

- Becoming a nursing home administrator
- Becoming an assisted living administrator
- Exploring a career in long term care
- Contacting the state licensing authority in each state
- Enrolling in college programs in each state
- Obtaining key publications in the long term care field
- Getting continuing education units

Dr. Allen can be reached via email through the website, or directly at jeallen@mindspring.com or jamesallen@unc.edu, or via phone(1-919-815-0387) or fax (1-919-933-6825).

Continuing education units for both nursing home and assisted living administrators are also available through the website (www.LongTermCareEducation.com).

*Springer also publishes similar text and exam review guides for assisted living administrators.*

*Visit Springer Publishing Company website to place inquiries or your order: www.springerpub.com*

# The Licensing Exam Review Guide in Nursing Home Administration

## Sixth Edition

*927 Test Questions in the*
*National Examination Format*
*on the NAB Domains of Practice*

**James E. Allen, PhD, MSPH, CNHA**
*Associate Professor of Health Policy and Administration, Emeritus*
*University of North Carolina at Chapel Hill*
*Chapel Hill, North Carolina*

SPRINGER PUBLISHING COMPANY
NEW YORK

Springer Publishing Company, LLC
11 West 42nd Street
New York, NY 10036
www.springerpub.com

*Acquisitions Editor:* Sheri W. Sussman
*Cover Design:* Steve Pisano
*Composition:* Newgen Imaging

ISBN: 978-0-8261-0706-0
E-book ISBN: 978-0-8261-0707-7
12 13/ 5 4 3

The author and the publisher of this Work have made every effort to use sources believed to
be reliable to provide information that is accurate and compatible with the standards generally
accepted at the time of publication. Because medical science is continually advancing, our
knowledge base continues to expand. Therefore, as new information becomes available, changes
in procedures become necessary. We recommend that the reader always consult current research
and specific institutional policies before performing any clinical procedure. The author and
publisher shall not be liable for any special, consequential, or exemplary damages resulting, in
whole or in part, from the readers' use of, or reliance on, the information contained in this book.
The publisher has no responsibility for the persistence or accuracy of URLs for external or third-
party Internet Web sites referred to in this publication and does not guarantee that any content
on such Web sites is, or will remain, accurate or appropriate.

Cataloging-in-Publication Data is available at the Library of Congress.

Printed in the United States of America by Hamilton Printing

# Contents

## DOMAINS OF PRACTICE

### PART 1: NAB DOMAIN: MANAGEMENT, GOVERNANCE, LEADERSHIP

# PART 6: FACILITY POLICIES

## Putting the System Together

# Introduction: Uses of This Study Guide for the NAB Domains of Practice

The review questions in this guide are intended for use by persons who are studying for the national licensure examination.

Sample study questions are provided here from several texts and sources in the long-term care field, including more than 70 questions on the Final Rules for Medicare and Medicaid Requirements for Long-Term Care Facilities (Appendix PP) and Nurse Aide Training and Competency Evaluation Programs.

National examination questions are picked by computer from a bank of more than 2,000 items. On average, more than 3,000 persons take this examination each year. Generally, about three unique exams are offered each year. The National Association of Boards of Examiners for Long-Term Care Administrators (NAB) exam is taken on a computer and each time the exam is taken the applicant will have a different set of questions unique to that exam.

# Format of the National Exam

The national examination is set up in the multiple choice, select the one best answer style of question to test the level of each candidate's knowledge.

This manual is designed to acquaint the user with relevant terms and provide practice in the multiple choice, one best answer examination format.

Two basic benefits are received: (1) feedback on comprehension of the terms and concepts in areas similar to those covered in the national examination and (2) experience with the multiple choice testing format used in the national exam.

Use of this manual without the text and similar sources achieves only initial knowledge about the field of nursing home administration. The bits and pieces of information obtained from these study questions are not a substitute for systematically studying the basic principles and information contained in the reading materials for Long Term Care Education (LTCE) 201 and 202 (www.LongTermCareEducation.com) and other equivalent resources.

# The "One Best Answer" Testing Format

There is always one best answer to each of the questions in this book. In the following question, only one answer can be correct.

The Lifespan Respite Care Act, allowing for the first time public payment to relatives to give care to family members, was passed in _____.

1. 1995
2. 2006
3. 2007
4. 2008

Because the Lifespan Respite Care Act was passed in 2006 (answer 2) all of the other answers are completely wrong.

In the following question, however, options 1, 2, and 4 are all partially correct, but 3 is the correct answer because it is the most complete (best) answer.

In the nursing facility a resident may perform services for the facility if the services are _____.

1. voluntary
2. paid at or above prevailing rates
3. in the plan of care
4. light duty in nature

All four options are partially correct, services performed must be voluntarily assumed, paid for at or above prevailing wage rates, and light duty in nature. However, even if services performed by a resident meet the three requirements in options 1, 2, and 4, they are prohibited if not in the resident's plan of care. Hence, 3 is the one best answer.

Following is an additional example.

Control is the evaluation by the organization decision makers of _____.

1. capital assets
2. the outputs of the organization
3. deficit spending
4. employee goals

The correct answer is 2, the outputs of the organization. Each of the other options is potentially correct. Organization decision makers *do* evaluate or make managerial judgments about capital assets, deficit spending if it occurs, and employee goals. However, the key word in the question is *control*. The correct answer is the answer that best defines control behavior by organizational decision makers. Answer 2 more fully defines control than any of the other three.

Sometimes the respondent is asked to mark the answer that is the least correct; for example:

The National Labor Relations Board does not _____.

1. determine what the bargaining units shall be
2. conduct representation elections by secret ballot
3. investigate unfair labor practices
4. make court decisions

The answer is 4. Answers 1, 2, and 3 are all activities the National Labor Relations Board *does do.*

# Deciding What the Question Is

A key to successfully answering multiple choice questions is correctly deciding what is being asked; for example:

> In states that still require government permission to build new nursing homes, if the health authority believes a shortage of beds exists, it may _____.

1. require that additional beds be built
2. let a contract for building new beds
3. advertise for bids
4. issue a permit to build (Certificate of Need)

The issue being tested here is, does the respondent know the functions and typical scope of powers exercised by a public health planning authority? The respondent needs to know that powers of health planning authorities are limited to granting permission for the applicant to build new beds.

To answer the question correctly, the respondent needs to further under-stand that local and state health planning authorities normally have no power to require that additional beds be built, to let contracts for building new beds, or to advertise for or let bids for constructing facilities with new beds. These are activities performed by the owners of the new facilities.

# Deciding What the Answer Is

Once the respondent has accurately decided *the question* about which he or she is being tested, the *one best answer* to the question must be selected. If the respondent knows what the answer ought to be, a useful technique is to look immediately for the correct answer; for example:

> For nursing facilities, meeting accreditation requirements set by the JCAHO (Joint Commission on Accreditation for Healthcare Organizations) is _____.
>
> 1. voluntary
> 2. mandatory
> 3. required to receive Medicaid payments
> 4. required to receive Medicare payments

If the reader knows that meeting requirements set by JCAHO is entirely voluntary for nursing facilities, he or she should look immediately for the correct answer, which in this case is 1. The other options can then be read to assure that there is not a better or more correct or complete option to mark as the correct answer.

To answer this question correctly the reader needs specific information: for example, knowledge of Medicare and Medicaid requirements for nursing facilities and the Federal requirements that must be met for reimbursement for Medicare or Medicaid patient charges. If read hastily, this question could be deceptive because *hospital* accreditation by JCAHO *is* required for hospital eligibility for reimbursement of Medicare patient charges. The equivalent for nursing homes is to meet the Federal requirements set by the Federal and state governments.

Thus, several areas of understanding may be tested simultaneously by a single question such as the one in this example.

# Strategies for Test Taking

Test taking, like driving a car, is an acquired skill. It is a complex task that, once learned, can become second nature when the techniques are established. In addition, practice in answering the types of questions that may be asked can ease the tension level when in the actual test situation. The following are some strategies for taking computer-based multiple-choice tests.

In an examination consisting of 150 questions, each with four possible answers, the reader must cycle through 600 possible answers. Giving equal energy to each of the 600 possible options can lead to mental fatigue early in the examination and may result in unintentional errors. Several *techniques* are available *to help reduce mental fatigue.*

## MARKING QUESTIONS FOR LATER REVIEW
The test will contain questions that the reader can answer with confidence, but there will inevitably be somewhere the answer is only a guess.

To save time and energy, it is advisable to proceed through the entire exam at a steady pace, marking for later review questions about which the reader is unsure.

Do not try to puzzle out each doubtful or unknown question in the order in which it appears. Go on to the next. This assures reasonably quick progress through the exam. Using this strategy, it will be found that a large proportion of questions will have been correctly answered during the first run-through. A second attempt to complete the remaining items will often reveal the answers at this stage.

## MAKING FINAL CHOICES
Once all items have been marked, it is time to return for a final decision about the choice made.

Experience has shown that the first answer chosen is often the best one. However, if the respondent is sure, on restudying the question, that a different response is the correct one, the answer originally marked should be changed.

## USING THE TIME AVAILABLE
The goal is to achieve the best possible score on the examination. For most people this should mean taking advantage of all of the time available. Rereading the questions and assuring oneself that the correct answer has been chosen is usually time well spent. In multiple-choice questions there is often *one key word or phrase* that may elude the reader on the first reading, but might change the answer dramatically.

## FINAL REVIEW
If there is time, the respondent should assure him or herself that the *question being asked* in every item has been correctly understood and the correct answer marked.

# Domains of Practice

# NAB Domain: Management, Governance, Leadership

# Learning How to Manage the Health Care Organization

Questions 1–31 portray often encountered situations in the nursing home profession. Rationale for answers to questions 1–31 can be found in the back of this book preceding the answer key.

Questions 32 and following flow sequentially through topics in *Nursing Home Administration,* 6th ed., by James E. Allen, MSPH, PhD, CNHA. Answers can be found on the page numbers in parentheses following each of these questions. In Part 6, answers can be found in *Nursing Home Administration,* 6th edition, and *Nursing Home Federal Requirements: Guidelines to Surveyors and Survey Protocols,* 7th edition, by James E. Allen (Springer Publishing Company). Those found in *Nursing Home Federal Requirements* are distinguished by the reference (see Federal Requirements App. P and PP).

1. The most likely single cause for the series of bankruptcies among larger nursing home chains around the year 2000 was ____.
   1. Too small increases in government reimbursement rates
   2. Paying too much for acquisitions in 1998 and 1999
   3. Not taking advantage of falling interest rates
   4. Thinking too small

2. In a chance conversation with the owner of an eight-facility chain, the newly hired administrator for the oldest facility in the chain indicates that, since the mortgage is fully retired, he will concentrate more on being effective than efficient since his Quality Indicators are all at or above his state's average. The owner would likely ____.
   1. Be pleased
   2. Be distressed
   3. Be content
   4. Praise the newly hired administrator

3. Occupancy of Facility A has been a steady 70% since Prospective Payment System was introduced. Two weeks ago, a new 120-bed equally equipped facility opened several blocks away. The Facility A administrator tells the admissions counselor to continue the usual recruitment approach. The chain owners ought to ____.
   1. Rest comfortably
   2. Seek a new administrator
   3. Appoint a new admissions counselor
   4. Take no action

4. Bankruptcies among larger nursing home chains prior to 2000 ____.
   1. Were frequent
   2. Were ubiquitous
   3. Were highly unusual
   4. Were routinely declared to avoid too much accumulated debt

5. Under the Prospective Payment System, nursing facilities' reimbursed costs _____.
   1. Were about the same as earlier
   2. Were more bundled
   3. Used an unbundled cost structure
   4. Were reimbursement for actual costs

6. In recent years Medicare has _____.
   1. Allowed facilities to make a modest profit
   2. Shifted more costs onto nursing facilities
   3. Eased up on economic pressures previously placed on facilities
   4. Remained relatively unchanged in its reimbursement structure

7. The nurse newly promoted to director of nurses (DON) insists on giving four RN hours of patient care each day on the Alzheimer's wing in the 175-bed facility. The administrator should _____.
   1. Praise the new DON for her resident-centeredness
   2. Appoint an assistant DON
   3. Adapt the job description to fit her pattern
   4. Seek a new DON

8. The applicant for the administrator position in a facility near a large teaching hospital who insists that, if hired, as before with his rural facility, he would not let the Medicare reimbursement policies affect his case mix _____.
   1. Should be hired
   2. Is likely to succeed if hired
   3. Can likely succeed in his goal
   4. Is out of touch

9. The newly hired assistant to the administrator insists the organizational chart line between his position and the Department of Nursing be a solid line. The administrator should _____.
   1. Agree in general
   2. Agree to this special case
   3. Ask the DON for his or her opinion
   4. Be forewarned

10. The medical supplies provider tells the administrator of a facility that has not paid bills the past 3 months, but is now operating under a bankruptcy judge's approved plan for restructuring, that no more deliveries will be made until past bills are fully paid. The medical supplies provider _____.
    1. Is smart to cut losses at that point
    2. Does not understand how bankruptcy works
    3. Will now likely get his past due bills paid
    4. Is farsighted

**11.** An administrator who adopts the management-by-walking-around (MBWA) approach by walking through the facility and intently observing weekly has _____.
1. Become an effective leader
2. Chosen a good management style
3. Failed to understand MBWA
4. Implemented a useful strategy

**12.** The nursing facility administrator who, using the management-by-walking-around (MBWA) technique, succeeds in actually making appropriate corrections on the spot during his rounds _____.
1. Is effectively implementing the concept
2. Gains additional power through the process
3. Exhibits appropriate leadership
4. Doesn't understand MBWA

**13.** The rate of increase in the total number of nursing facilities in the United States during the years 2008–2012 is _____.
1. Likely to be about level
2. Likely to double
3. Likely to triple to accommodate the baby boomer generation
4. Likely to decrease markedly

**14.** The applicant for administrator of the facility insists that he has successfully used democratic leadership to the exclusion of all other leadership styles. The interviewer should _____.
1. Recommend hiring this candidate
2. Praise the candidate
3. Be favorably impressed
4. Continue to interview candidates

**15.** The candidate for administrator said she used a variety of administrative styles, but couldn't say exactly which she would use in every circumstance. The interviewer should be _____.
1. Favorably impressed
2. Unfavorably impressed
3. Concerned about possible indecisiveness
4. Looking for one leadership style

**16.** The candidate for administrator indicated that she consistently chooses the charismatic style of leadership. This should _____ the interviewer.
1. Reassure
2. Alert
3. Confirm the candidate's qualifications to
4. Please

**17.** The costs of providing subacute care to nursing home residents _____.
1. Is perhaps triple that of the more typical patient
2. Covered by Medicare
3. Absorbed by Medicaid if Medicare coverage is inadequate
4. Mostly covered by private insurance

**18.** The nurse supervisor who had just been appointed DON announced at the first department head meeting that she had circulated a memo among the nurses that only formal communications were to be allowed in the nursing department. The administrator should _____.
1. Be relieved
2. Confirm the decision
3. Be supportive
4. Anticipate problems

**19.** The department head was not surprised to learn that the employee had only heard his positive comments to the employee and ignored his criticisms. The department head's grasp of the communication process is _____.
1. Deficient
2. Appropriate
3. Out of focus
4. Inadequate

**20.** The administrator routinely accepted as his nearly exclusive information source the director of nursing's positive reports on how nursing was going well. The administrator is _____.
1. Showing appropriate confidence in the DON
2. Utilizing the DON properly
3. Realizing a successful appointment has been made
4. Placing him at risk

**21.** Periodic shortage of nurses available for nursing home employment _____.
1. Is being solved by community college programs
2. Is decreasing
3. Can be readily solved by hiring temporary nurses
4. Is likely to remain for the foreseeable future

**22.** Congress and the federal rule makers behave as if the facility will run successfully if Congress and Centers for Medicare and Medicaid Services can write enough rules. They are _____.
1. Incorrect
2. Correct, according to behavior theory
3. Pessimistic about the need for rules
4. Correct, according to emerging management theory

**23.** When the administrator notices that the DON seeks to turn as many duties as possible over to housekeeping, the administrator should conclude that the DON is _____.
1. Behaving normally
2. Holding a grudge against housekeeping
3. Unwilling to be cooperative
4. Wielding power desirably

**24.** The administrator insists that a timely copy of all reports generated within the facility come across her desk before anyone signs them. The administrator is _____.
1. Not rationalizing her management information system
2. Making appropriate and desirable requests
3. Exercising good judgment
4. Initiating an appropriate management information system

25. The administrator notices that incident reports are being insufficiently filled out, but does nothing, believing that the situation will likely correct itself. The administrator is _____.
    1. Practicing effective control
    2. Likely to be correct
    3. Failing to control effectively
    4. Right to monitor the situation for a period of time

26. Corporate sends a directive to its flagship facility administrator, directing the administrator's attention more toward outcome of resident care than cost of resident care during the coming 12 months. Corporate is more concerned with _____ than with _____.
    1. Effectiveness/efficiency
    2. Efficiency/effectiveness
    3. Expenses/inputs
    4. Expenses/throughput

27. The long-term care sector receiving increased funding and attention from the federal government is the _____.
    1. Home health care sector
    2. Volunteer hospice group association
    3. Long-term care hospital sector
    4. Private insurance industry

28. The concept that nursing homes should be reimbursed by states for their actual costs was part of the _____.
    1. Emerging Medicare approach
    2. Federal administration's goal as seen in new budgetary appropriations
    3. Hatch Amendment
    4. Goal statements of most state governments

29. The intense health care cost-shifting efforts among providers such as Medicare, Medicaid, and local governments is _____.
    1. On the wane
    2. Likely to continue
    3. Leading to increased reimbursements
    4. Good for the nursing home profession

30. Worried about the level of actual resident care being achieved in the facility, the administrator directs the nurses to spend less time charting and more time focusing on the effectiveness of care being given to residents. The likely result will be _____.
    1. Better resident care, possibly increased deficiency citations
    2. Better resident care, decreased deficiency citations
    3. No real improvement in resident care, decreased charting
    4. Greater sensitivity to resident need and better documentation

31. The new social worker informs the head of nursing that admissions is all she has time for and that nursing must monitor and document each resident's socio-psychological experiences. The new social worker is _____.
    1. Responding appropriately to priorities
    2. Achieving a better balance of assignments within the facility
    3. Responding inappropriately
    4. Likely to improve the case mix dramatically

**32.** Attempting to find the right person for each well-defined job is known as the management function of _____. (pp. 2–5)
1. Personnel work
2. Interviewing
3. Staffing
4. The job search

**33.** The administrator who takes steps that assure the goals are accomplished and that each job is done as planned is successfully _____. (pp. 2–5)
1. Getting results
2. Improving outputs
3. Controlling quality
4. Sensing organizational needs

**34.** The administrator's job is to assure that the _____ employees do the tasks of the organization at an acceptable quality level. (pp. 2–5)
1. Best prepared
2. Trained
3. Appropriate
4. Unmotivated

**35.** The administrator who conducts a national search for a director of nursing position and interviews 20 candidates from 7 different surrounding states by phone is engaged in the managerial function of _____. (pp. 2–5)
1. Directing personnel development
2. Staffing
3. Broad personnel searches
4. In-depth interviewing

**36.** In the end, it can be said that the administrator's responsibility to meet resident care needs and facility financial needs are _____. (pp. 2–5)
1. Clearly unequal
2. A mismatch
3. Both about equal
4. Unclear

**37.** Superior performance depends on taking exceptional care of residents via superior service and _____. (pp. 2–5)
1. Constant attention to the bottom line
2. Constant innovation
3. Attention to detail
4. A good attitude

**38.** Superior performance for a nursing facility comes through _____. (pp. 2–5)
1. Having all the beds full
2. Achieving consistent profitability
3. Innovation in ways to serve residents
4. Efficient management of the budget

**39.** The superb nursing facility is superb by virtue of its _____. (pp. 2–5)
1. Success in attention to consistent profitability
2. Success in serving the residents
3. Reputation in the community as a friendly place
4. Achieving superior ratings

40. Answering the phones and resident call bells with common courtesy and doing things that work are examples of _____. (pp. 2–5)
    1. Good sense
    2. Uncommon perceptions
    3. An ability to be practical
    4. A blinding flash of the obvious

41. Giving every employee the space to innovate at least a little; listening to residents and acting on their ideas; and wandering around with residents, staff, and suppliers are examples of the difficult-to-achieve _____. (pp. 2–5)
    1. Long-range goals
    2. Short-range goals
    3. Common sense, obvious
    4. Typical facility approach

## 1.1.1 LEVELS OF MANAGEMENT

42. In a facility of 120 beds, the administrator _____ personally perform each of the management tasks. (pp. 5–7)
    1. Need not
    2. Should
    3. Over a month will
    4. Over a year will

43. To assure that all the management tasks are successfully accomplished, the administrator of a 120-bed facility will typically divide management into _____. (pp. 5–7)
    1. Two layers
    2. Three layers
    3. Eight cooperating teams
    4. Four teams

44. A licensed person responsible for formulating and enforcing policies that will be applied to an entire facility is thought of as a/an _____. (pp. 5–7)
    1. Upper-level manager
    2. Senior administrator
    3. Board member
    4. Owner

45. The staff member responsible for reporting to upper-level management and at the same time interacting significantly with several lower-level managers is the _____. (pp. 5–7)
    1. Director of finance
    2. Director of nursing
    3. Charge nurse
    4. Assistant to the administrator

**46.** The staff person for whom both upward and downward communication skills are the most necessary is the _____. (pp. 5–7)
1. Staff development coordinator
2. Director of nursing
3. Nursing supervisor
4. Assistant administrator for personnel

**47.** When the director of nursing makes an effective policy decision without consulting the administrator, that impacts all nursing personnel, the administrator should _____. (pp. 5–7)
1. Be pleased
2. Nevertheless be somewhat concerned
3. Counsel with the director of nursing about chain of command
4. Begin the search for a new director of nursing

**48.** In the typical nursing facility, the decision-making process is _____ establishment of lower, middle, and upper levels of management. (pp. 5–7)
1. Noticeably more complicated than the simple
2. Normally accomplished by the
3. Successful if the ownership assures effective
4. Rendered relatively uncomplicated through

## 1.1.2 LINE–STAFF RELATIONSHIPS

**49.** Among the following positions, the _____ has no authority to make decisions for the facility. (pp. 7–8)
1. Director of nursing
2. Supply room manager
3. Assistant to the administrator
4. Evening charge nurse

**50.** Decisions made by persons on the staff to whom the administrator has delegated line authority are, in the final analysis, regarded as decisions by _____. (pp. 7–8)
1. The owners
2. The board of directors
3. The administrator
4. The department head holding such line authority

**51.** When a nurse practitioner, who is more highly qualified than the director of nursing, gives orders to nurses in the hallways, the director of nurses should feel _____. (pp. 7–8)
1. Reaffirmed
2. Undermined
3. That quality of care is being reinforced
4. That a useful support system is functioning

**52.** In times of crisis, corporate representatives, who hold a staff or advisory relationship to their counterparts in the local facility, may expect that their advice as staff be _____. (pp. 7–8)
  1. Regarded as strong recommendations
  2. Approached on a "take or leave it" basis
  3. Respected
  4. Acted on as carrying line authority

# 1.2
# Forecasting

**53.** As a generalization, it can be asserted that managerial success belongs to those who _____. (pp. 9–11)
  1. Successfully prepare for the future
  2. Are reactive on every front
  3. Constantly take initiatives
  4. Conserve resources

**54.** Nursing home administrators should anticipate and successfully prepare for _____. (pp. 9–11)
  1. Increased reimbursement
  2. New long-term care legislation
  3. Increased longevity
  4. Rapid change

**55.** The long-term care industry has entered a period in which _____ change(s) can be expected. (pp. 9–11)
  1. Fewer
  2. More dramatic
  3. Rapid and far reaching
  4. A more controlled rate of

**56.** The ability to accurately predict the future implications for nursing facilities of new trends to which the present environment may offer small clues is the skill needed to successfully _____. (pp. 9–11)
  1. Forecast
  2. Review
  3. Read the meaning of history
  4. Learn from the past

**57.** Historically, during the 1970s and early 1980s (until the diagnosis related group method of reimbursement, i.e., the DRGs) nursing facility administrators made long-range projections during a period of _____. (pp. 9–11)
  1. Unlimited change
  2. Intense social scrutiny of reimbursement mechanisms
  3. Relative stability in the health care field
  4. Rapid social change

**58.** The rate of change in the health care field is believed to be _____. (pp. 9–11)
1. Slowing down
2. Coming under control
3. Increasing exponentially
4. Retrenching

**59.** Researchers have predicted that every 10 years _____ of all current knowledge and accepted practices in the health care and other industries will be _____. (pp. 9–11)
1. One-fourth/obsolete
2. One-half/obsolete
3. Three-fourths/still usable
4. Four-fifths/still usable

**60.** It is conceivable that the core business of the nursing home in this decade will _____ the core business of the nursing home of the next decade. (pp. 9–11)
1. Be entirely different from
2. Remain relatively stable and closely resemble
3. Undergo change at a slower pace than
4. Be remarkably similar to

**61.** One should expect that over the next few decades the rules governing the nursing home will be _____. (pp. 9–11)
1. Relatively stable
2. New, never experienced before
3. Even more formalized by Congressional legislation
4. Enforced less due to decreased personnel available to state and federal agencies

**62.** Nursing homes that stick to conventional formulas for success are/will _____. (pp. 9–11)
1. Be more likely to survive
2. Miss new markets and be in a backwash
3. Be more likely to produce a steady profit
4. Survive while those introducing constant change will lose needed focus

**63.** In the text it is argued that for the first time in human history the capacity exists to provide _____. (pp. 9–11)
1. Complete health care for all citizens
2. A high level of health care for all citizens
3. More health care than any nation can afford
4. Affordable health care for all

**64.** The roles possible for hospitals, nursing homes, home health agencies, and managed care organizations are _____. (pp. 9–11)
1. Predictable and, likely, manageable
2. Sorting themselves out
3. Being more and more successfully managed by government
4. Endless and will remain up for grabs

**65.** The staff in nursing facilities, over the next two decades, will likely _____. (pp. 9–11)
1. Experience culture shock
2. Be reduced in staff/patient ratios
3. Become accustomed to a predictable core business
4. Remain committed to the facility, lowering turnover

# 1.3
# Planning

## 1.3.1 WHY PLAN?

**66.** Plans can best be said to be statements of the _____. (pp. 11–15)
  *1.* Hopes of the administrator
  *2.* Hopes of the ownership
  *3.* Prediction of the next steps needed
  *4.* Organizational goals of the facility

**67,** In order to survive, each facility must _____. (pp. 11–15)
  *1.* Deal with the outside world
  *2.* Have immeasurably more income than expenses
  *3.* Know what the future will bring years in advance
  *4.* Write enough policies to cover all contingencies

**68.** A major advantage associated with carefully developed plans is making it possible to _____. (pp. 11–15)
  *1.* Control the future
  *2.* Not repeat past mistakes
  *3.* Compare what happens to what was predicted
  *4.* Compare what happens to past experiences

**69.** When external conditions change, plans _____. (pp. 11–15)
  *1.* Should remain in place
  *2.* Can be altered to meet the changed conditions
  *3.* Should be monitored, but not radically altered
  *4.* Are of decreased value

**70.** The observation about the idea that "if it ain't broke, don't fix it" is _____. (pp. 11–15)
  *1.* That this is functionally valuable conventional wisdom
  *2.* That if it ain't broke today, it will be tomorrow
  *3.* That too few managers understand this good advice
  *4.* That this is a solid insight one can depend upon

**71.** The approach to planning known as SWOT refers to focusing on _____. (pp. 11–15)
  *1.* Strengths, weaknesses, occupancy level, and threats
  *2.* Strategies, weaknesses, opportunities, and threats
  *3.* Strengths, weaknesses, opportunities, and threats
  *4.* Statistics, work options, opportunities, and trends

## 1.3.2 STEPS IN PLANNING

72. When considering building a new facility, necessary approvals by government agencies, such as zoning requirements, building codes, certificate of need, is/are _____. (pp. 11–15)
    1. Routinely issued to applicants
    2. Sometimes difficult or impossible to obtain
    3. Available to all applicants
    4. Reserved for certain applicants

73. Looking at competitors' expansion plans, occupancy levels, and local hospital plans when considering building a nursing facility is known as conducting a _____. (pp. 11–15)
    1. Needs assessment
    2. Review
    3. Constructive analysis
    4. Construction review

74. When planning a new nursing facility, the goal of being in operation within four months is best described as a/an _____. (pp. 11–15)
    1. Unrealistic goal
    2. Long-range objective
    3. Short-range objective
    4. Realistic goal

75. As a general rule, the planning process moves from _____. (pp. 11–15)
    1. Goal to goal
    2. Unrealistic to realistic
    3. General to specific
    4. Vague to sharp

76. One mentioned view of the planning process includes the observation that _____. (pp. 11–15)
    1. The future will change our plans
    2. Keeping to a carefully thought-out plan is essential
    3. Planning produces a reasonable degree of certainty
    4. Plans, once in place, keep us on track toward our goal

77. Nursing home administrators who expect the unexpected and thrive on it _____. (pp. 11–15)
    1. Exhibit an unnecessary anxiety about the future
    2. Are too pessimistic
    3. Will last in the profession
    4. Will not make enough plans

78. The area offering the richest opportunities for innovation is _____. (pp. 11–15)
    1. Nursing
    2. Financing
    3. The unexpected
    4. Clear new trends

**79.** When one accepts the idea that change is a permanent part of life _____. (pp. 11–15)
1. Life becomes more uncontrollable
2. Life becomes less comfortable
3. Uncertainty proliferates
4. One can take advantage of new opportunities

**80.** One must assume that other nursing home administrators in the community _____. (pp. 11–15)
1. Have found the best ways to "climb the mountain"
2. Are excellent marketers
3. May fail, if you fail
4. Are "searching for new ways to climb the mountain"

# 1.4
# Organizing

**81.** In the process of organizing the work of a facility, it is of real importance to assure that _____. (pp. 16–25)
1. Workers are satisfied
2. Any union preferences are met
3. There is no duplication of work
4. Sufficient managers are appointed

**82.** Organizing is the first step in implementation of a/an _____. (pp. 16–25)
1. Challenge to the workers
2. Plan
3. Organizational chart
4. Organizational reorganization

**83.** What the worker does, how the worker does it, what aids are necessary, what is accomplished, and what skills are needed are parts of a _____. (pp. 16–25)
1. Job family
2. Job review
3. Needs assessment
4. Job analysis

**84.** It can be argued that all nursing facility administrators organize their facility according to _____. (pp. 16–25)
1. Local requirements
2. The owners' needs
3. Some theory of organization
4. The same theory of organization

**85.** Viewing organizations as systems has the advantage of offering the manager a framework for visualizing the _____ of the organization. (pp. 16–25)
1. Inputs
2. Outputs
3. Internal and external environment
4. Restraints

**86.** An organized or complex whole, an assembling or combining of things or parts forming a complex or single whole, best describes the _____. (pp. 16–25)
1. Systems concept
2. Organizational theory concept
3. Complexity concept
4. Organizational chart concept

**87.** A primary advantage of systems theory is that it serves as a tool for making sense of the world by making clearer _____. (pp. 16–25)
1. How people interact
2. Interrelationships within and outside the organization
3. Interrelationships among the staff
4. Interactions between staff and residents and their responsible parties

**88.** If the outputs of the organization do not meet the administrator's expectation he takes _____ actions to bring the outputs into line with those planned. (pp. 16–25)
1. Results-oriented
2. Quick
3. Effective
4. Control

**89.** In essence, what nursing facilities do is use money to hire staff and provide materials needed to _____. (pp. 16–25)
1. Give patient care
2. Show profitability
3. Achieve conformity to regulations
4. Meet owner requirements

**90.** The patient care that is given by the facility (i.e., the output) _____. (pp. 16–25)
1. Is usually good
2. Can range from good to unacceptable
3. Achieved cures for the residents
4. Meets federal and state requirements

**91.** Asking if the work accomplished by the facility is up to expected standards and, if not, taking corrective actions is the act of _____. (pp. 16–25)
1. Taking charge
2. Reviewing results
3. Controlling quality
4. Control of the inputs

92. The administrator uses _____ as the guidelines to compare the output with the expected results. (pp. 16–25)
    1. The facility's policies and plans of action
    2. Goals
    3. Stated objectives
    4. External judgments

93. The passage of the Nursing Home Reform Act of 1987 can be viewed as a form of _____ the nursing home industry. (pp. 16–25)
    1. Oppressive measure imposed on
    2. Object-oriented programming goals for
    3. External feedback of
    4. Internal feedback of

94. The external environment of the nursing facility consists of _____. (pp. 16–25)
    1. Opportunities
    2. Available initiatives
    3. Constraints
    4. Opportunities and constraints

95. If something relates meaningfully to a nursing facility, but is something over which the facility has no control, for example, enforcement of the federal certification requirements, it can be said to be _____. (pp. 16–25)
    1. Outside the facility's environment
    2. A constriction to the facility being successful
    3. A constraint in the external environment
    4. An opportunity

96. Increasing availability of managed care contracts, new niches, and increasing numbers of elderly needing care can be considered to be _____. (pp. 16–25)
    1. Constraints
    2. Changes
    3. Opportunities
    4. Additional requirements

97. Systems analysis is most/equally useful to _____. (pp. 16–25)
    1. The administrator
    2. The director of nursing
    3. The head of housekeeping
    4. The administrator, director of nursing, and head of housekeeping

98. Typically, the output of the nursing home as a system becomes the input for _____. (pp. 16–25)
    1. Psychiatric hospitals
    2. Managed care organizations
    3. Health maintenance organizations
    4. The hospital or the resident's home

99. A nursing home and similar organizations can grow _____. (pp. 16–25)
    1. Within a limited time span
    2. Until negative entropy applies
    3. Until resources run low
    4. Without any time limit

**100.** The entropy process is considered a universal law of nature that all organisms _____. (pp. 16–25)
1. Can grow indefinitely
2. Move toward death
3. Can expand
4. Can expand as long as more inputs are available

**101.** As a general characteristic of organizations, it has been argued that, in general, organizations seek to _____. (pp. 16–25)
1. Grow
2. Maintain their current size
3. Shrink as needed
4. Be flexible in adapting to change

**102.** Once in place, organizations become creatures of habit and develop a tendency to _____ change. (pp. 16–25)
1. Embrace
2. Resist
3. Build on
4. Create

**103.** The most predictable response of a nursing facility experiencing a "disruptive employee" is to _____. (pp. 16–25)
1. Hold an inservice
2. Counsel with the employee
3. Let the employee go
4. Contact the EEOC and ask for action

**104.** When a nursing facility chain goes from being the leader to being behind the pack, this can likely be attributed to _____. (pp. 16–25)
1. Bullheadedness of top management
2. Overconfidence
3. Lack of enthusiasm
4. A deep reservoir of outmoded attitudes and policies

**105.** The training received in nursing school, medical school, and physical therapy school tends to _____. (pp. 16–25)
1. Create resistance to change
2. Encourage innovation
3. Open graduates to change
4. Focus on niches

**106.** The real purpose of systems thinking is to _____. (pp. 16–25)
1. Empower people to introduce organizational change
2. Ensure that the current adjustments remain
3. Tutor employees in how the organization is arranged
4. Achieve conformity to the organizational chart

**107.** The movement of American medicine from 80% general practitioners in 1870 to 20% general practitioners in the 1990s is an illustration of the tendency of organizations to _____. (pp. 16–25)
   *1.* Grow increasingly complex
   *2.* Embrace change
   *3.* Reverse their ratios
   *4.* Achieve independence

# 1.6
# Directing

**108.** Directing is the process of communicating to employees what is to be done by each of them and _____. (p. 27)
   *1.* Enforcing the rules
   *2.* Rewriting the rules
   *3.* Helping them to accomplish it
   *4.* Providing active training courses

## 1.6.1 POLICY MAKING

**109.** It is _____ to make policies that direct the activities of employees everywhere in the facility 24 hours a day. (pp. 27–32)
   *1.* Impossible
   *2.* Improbable
   *3.* Possible
   *4.* Undesirable

**110.** It is neither possible nor desirable to establish policies for _____. (pp. 27–32)
   *1.* All nursing assistants
   *2.* The admissions coordinator
   *3.* Every conceivable situation
   *4.* Situations with some variability

**111.** The specific spelling out, step by step, of the intended implementation of a policy is known as a _____. (pp. 27–32)
   *1.* Set of controls
   *2.* Detailing of policy
   *3.* Set of procedures
   *4.* Set of limits

**112.** A detailed plan of actions expected of each employee upon hearing the fire alarm is known as _____. (pp. 27–32)
1. A clearly developed policy
2. A set of procedures
3. Management expectations
4. Detailed instructions

## 1.6.2 DECISION MAKING

**113.** The internal process by which managers make decisions is _____. (p. 32)
1. Well understood
2. A subject of little interest
3. Entirely subjective
4. Imprecise, not well understood

**114.** It is the administrator's job to assure that all employees make the right decisions for the facility _____. (p. 32)
1. In every case
2. With a minimum of worry
3. Quickly
4. As often as possible

## 1.6.3 LEADERSHIP

**115.** Organizations that thrive over an extended period of time depend on having _____. (p. 33)
1. Large profit margins
2. Charismatic leadership
3. Consistent leadership
4. Effective leaders

**116.** Compared to defining the concept *deciding,* defining the concept *leading* is _____. (p. 33)
1. Less difficult
2. More difficult
3. Equally difficult
4. Researched and understood

**117.** The concept that history is *made* or measurably influenced by individuals who become leaders is known as _____. (p. 33)
1. Leadership by men
2. Leadership by innovators
3. The great leadership theory of history
4. Man, the maker theory

**118.** Democratic, authoritarian, and laissez-faire are _____. (p. 34)
1. Types of leadership styles
2. Outmoded models for today's leaders
3. Discounted today
4. Types of political positions

**119.** A supervising staff member the administrator might most want to provide leadership by walking around is the _____. (pp. 34–35)
1. Receptionist
2. Charge nurse
3. Director of nursing
4. Director of housekeeping

**120.** A major information advantage to leadership by walking around is the opportunity to _____. (p. 35)
1. Check on staff
2. Engage in naive listening
3. Get out of the office
4. Check the floors

**121.** It is _____ to maintain the chain of command when an administrator practices managing by walking around. (p. 35)
1. Especially difficult
2. Especially easy
3. Entirely feasible
4. Impossible

**122.** The administrator's work begins once the ownership has set forth the _____ of the organization. (p. 39)
1. Full rules
2. Day-to-day rules and regulations
3. Mission statement
4. Procedures to be followed

**123.** The best time for the administrator to introduce change in the facility is when _____. (p. 35)
1. Everyone is ready for it
2. It is clear to all that the situation demands it
3. It will improve the bottom line
4. She doesn't have to

**124.** The better administrator is the one who _____. (pp. 35–37)
1. Spends most hours in the facility wings
2. In the administrator's office constantly explores ways to lead
3. Reviews reports as the primary information channel about the facility
4. Prepares for certification and the state to come in

**125.** For every successful decision the administrator makes, _____. (p. 35)
1. The administrator is praised
2. Recognition comes from those affected
3. He may experience one or two wipe-outs
4. Ownership is grateful

**126.** One thing the successful administrator remembers about the environment is that it _____. (p. 36)
1. Remains beyond control
2. Can be harnessed
3. Can be brought under control
4. Can be static

**127.** One reason for the administrator not to give all attention to the most immediate opportunity is that _____. (p. 36)
1. Corporate is unlikely to approve
2. Change costs too much energy
3. Better opportunities may also exist
4. It may not be what it seems

**128.** The best time to begin a move toward introducing a change into a facility is when _____. (p. 36)
1. Change is still on the horizon
2. Change is imminent
3. The climate is right
4. The staff are receptive

**129.** The "waves of change" that were encountered in the late 1990s are _____. (p. 36)
1. Getting more manageable
2. Coming slower, but are larger
3. Remaining somewhat static since the year 2000
4. Coming in set after set and getting bigger

**130.** In the views of some contemporary corporate managers, change should be viewed more as a/an _____. (pp. 35–37)
1. Continuous process, not an event
2. Process with some consistency
3. Predictable process that can be managed
4. Opportunity to consolidate past gains

**131.** Being knowledgeable about the field and having competence and experience will take today's administrator to _____. (p. 37)
1. Excellence
2. Good
3. The highest level
4. Charismatic leadership

**132.** When a nursing facility administrator has "that particular thing" in her blood she has a fire in the heart for _____. (p. 37)
1. Continuous quality improvement
2. Continuously improving the quality of daily life of each resident
3. A successful career
4. Being totally professional

**133.** Manager-centered leadership retains a _____ degree of control and uses _____ extensively. (p. 37)
1. Low/authority
2. Medium/authority
3. High/authority
4. High/charisma

**134.** Permitting the subordinates to make the decision and function within the limits defined by the manager is closest to a _____ style of management. (p. 37)
1. Laissez-faire
2. Democratic
3. Authoritarian
4. Charismatic

**135.** When deciding what style of management to employ in a given situation, the administrator should consider factors within himself, factors in the employees, and factors in the _____. (p. 38)
1. Organization
2. External environment
3. Five-year plan
4. One-year plan

**136.** A manager who is responsible for the development of more specific policies that interpret administration's policies for the employees one supervises is closest to _____ managing. (p. 39)
1. Upper-level
2. Middle-level
3. Lower-level
4. Integrated

**137.** The charge nurse responsible for applying policies provided by the director of nursing services is functioning most nearly at the _____ level of management. (p. 39)
1. Upper
2. Middle
3. Lower
4. Integrated

**138.** Origination: change, creation, and elimination of structure is the responsibility of _____ management. (p. 39)
1. Upper-level
2. Middle-level
3. Lower-level
4. Functional

**139.** Interpolation: supplementing and piecing out structure for the organization is the responsibility of _____ management. (p. 39)
1. Upper-level
2. Middle-level
3. Lower-level
4. Functional

**140.** Operational use of existing structure is the responsibility of _____ management. (p. 39)
 *1.* Upper-level
 *2.* Middle-level
 *3.* Lower-level
 *4.* Functional

**141.** According to Tannenbaum, the successful leader needs to be keenly aware of relevant forces in the situation, to understand herself, and also _____ vis-à-vis the situation. (p. 40)
 *1.* Be calm and purposeful
 *2.* Interpret successfully
 *3.* Have insight
 *4.* Be able to behave appropriately

**142.** The acts of the _____ leader are typically unexamined. (p. 40)
 *1.* Accepted
 *2.* Venerated
 *3.* Charismatic
 *4.* Fully established

## 1.6.4 POWER AND AUTHORITY

**143.** When one is able to motivate someone to do something he would not otherwise do, that person is said to be wielding _____. (p. 42)
 *1.* Undue influence
 *2.* Self-control
 *3.* Power
 *4.* Excessive influence

**144.** In the American culture power is a/an _____. (p. 42)
 *1.* Relatively well understood concept
 *2.* Accepted tradition for all members of society
 *3.* Complex concept
 *4.* Simple set of beliefs

**145.** The administrator's ability to award or withhold a year-end bonus represents _____ power held by the administrator. (p. 43)
 *1.* Punishment
 *2.* Overarching
 *3.* Financial
 *4.* Reward

**146.** Fear that the administrator may write a negative report and place it in one's personnel file represents the administrator's _____ power. (p. 43)
 *1.* Expert
 *2.* Personnel
 *3.* Controlling
 *4.* Punishment

**147.** Employees identifying and admiring the administrator yields _____ power to the administrator. (p. 43)
  *1.* Expert
  *2.* Exceptional
  *3.* Additional
  *4.* Referent

**148.** Two types of power available to all staff members are _____. (p. 44)
  *1.* Legitimate and reward
  *2.* Punishment and reward
  *3.* Referent and reward
  *4.* Expert and referent

**149.** As a general rule, it is better if an administrator can possess and exercise _____ power. (p. 44)
  *1.* Expert and referent
  *2.* Charismatic and punishment
  *3.* Expert and punishment
  *4.* Legitimate and punishment

**150.** The presence of numerous professions such as the medical, nursing, dental, and pharmaceutical professions in the facility tend to _____ the administrator's power. (p. 44)
  *1.* Constrain
  *2.* Increase
  *3.* Augment
  *4.* Supplement

## 1.6.5 COMMUNICATION SKILLS

**151.** Communication is the exchange of information and the transmission of _____. (p. 45)
  *1.* Meaning
  *2.* Memos of documentation
  *3.* Faxes
  *4.* Internet messages

**152.** The administrator initiates a communication and it is transmitted from its source to its destination. Communication has _____. (p. 46)
  *1.* Not yet taken place
  *2.* Been accomplished
  *3.* Been reviewed
  *4.* Been retrieved

**153.** Listening with intensity, acceptance, empathy, and a willingness to assume responsibility for understanding the speaker's complete message is sometimes called _____. (p. 46)
  *1.* Passive listening
  *2.* Attentive listening
  *3.* Active listening
  *4.* Paying full attention

**154.** Two systems of communication usually exist side by side in an organization and are known as _____. (p. 46)
    *1.* Active and inactive
    *2.* Upward and lateral
    *3.* First layer and second layer
    *4.* Formal and informal

**155.** Two nurses chatting while on break in the nurse's lounge about a patient's status is _____ communication. (p. 46)
    *1.* Upward
    *2.* Downward
    *3.* Horizontal
    *4.* Peer

**156.** Two nurses chatting about the most recent events in the administrator's office while on break in the nurses' lounge are engaged in _____ communication. (p. 46)
    *1.* Formal
    *2.* Informal
    *3.* Casual
    *4.* Gossip-type

**157.** It can be reasonably argued that every communication is likely to have _____. (p. 46)
    *1.* Intended impact
    *2.* Unintended consequences
    *3.* Serendipitous results
    *4.* Multiple levels of meaning

**158.** The informal communication process most closely resembles _____. (p. 46)
    *1.* The consultant pharmacist reporting findings to the director of nursing
    *2.* The nurse assistant chatting with a resident while making the bed
    *3.* The administrator calling a report in to corporate
    *4.* The charge nurse reporting to the nurse supervisor

**159.** The director of nursing giving instructions to the nurse supervisor is considered _____. (p. 46)
    *1.* Upward communication
    *2.* Downward communication
    *3.* Flawed communication
    *4.* To be done twice each shift

**160.** The nurse assistant reporting to the nurse supervisor about an incident in a patient room is an example of _____ communication. (p. 46)
    *1.* Upward
    *2.* Downward
    *3.* Optional
    *4.* Well-organized

**161.** The closer one gets to the organization center of control, the administrator's office, for example, the _____. (p. 46)
    *1.* More pronounced the emphasis on the exchange of information
    *2.* Less important constant information exchange becomes
    *3.* Less necessary written reports become
    *4.* More comfortably the administrator can operate

162. The nurse assistant, preoccupied and angry over unsettled matters at home, interprets the comments by the nurse as hostile comments. This illustrates a barrier to communication known as _____. (pp. 46–48)
    1. Differences in knowledge level
    2. Subgroup allegiance
    3. Status distance
    4. Agenda carrying

163. The charge nurse who remembers the words of praise from the director of nursing, but ignores the criticisms also received from the director of nursing illustrates a barrier to communication known as _____. (pp. 46–48)
    1. Selective hearing
    2. Subgroup allegiance
    3. Status distance
    4. Agenda carrying

164. The nurse assistant realizes that her fellow nurse assistant is sleeping much of the night shift, but decides not to rat on her. This illustrates _____. (pp. 46–48)
    1. Differences in knowledge level
    2. Subgroup allegiance
    3. Status distance
    4. The filter effect

165. The nurses aide realized the patient's condition should be pointed out to the attending physician who had just popped into the patient's room, but hesitated to approach the physician. This illustrates the effects of _____. (pp. 46–48)
    1. Differences in knowledge level
    2. Subgroup allegiance
    3. Status distance
    4. The filter effect

166. The medication nurse thought she understood what the pharmacist had just said about the side effects of a medication, but found the technical jargon used by the pharmacist to be intimidating. This illustrates _____. (pp. 46–48)
    1. Differences in knowledge level
    2. The language barrier
    3. Status distance
    4. The filter effect

167. The charge nurse decided not to write up an incident on her shift because four incidents had already been written up that week on her shift. This illustrates _____. (pp. 46–48)
    1. Differences in knowledge level
    2. Subgroup allegiance
    3. Self-protection
    4. The filter effect

**168.** The new 30-page-long policy on universal precautions contained so many new requirements that staff soon began to revert to their time-tested approaches in conducting patient care. This illustrates _____. (pp. 46–48)
   *1.* Differences in knowledge level
   *2.* Information overload
   *3.* Status distance
   *4.* The filter effect

## 1.6.6 ORGANIZATIONAL NORMS AND VALUES

**169.** Under Tag F241 the government defines dignity as caring for residents in a manner that maintains full recognition of the resident's _____. (pp. 49–50)
   *1.* Individuality
   *2.* Personal tastes
   *3.* Past types of activities
   *4.* Reasonable expectations

**170.** Dignity has been interpreted by states' examiners _____. (p. 50)
   *1.* With wide variations
   *2.* Fairly consistently
   *3.* Differently depending on the section of the country
   *4.* With excellent consistency

**171.** Standardized patterns of required behaviors developed by the facility to enable staff to accomplish necessary work defines a _____. (p. 49)
   *1.* Norm
   *2.* Set of values
   *3.* Specific patterns
   *4.* Role

**172.** Over the years 1999 and 2008 the percentage of nursing facilities in the United States given deficiencies in Quality of Life, dignity _____. (p. 49)
   *1.* Held steady
   *2.* Went consistently up
   *3.* Varied widely by state and over time
   *4.* Went lower as facilities improved care

**173.** Treating all residents with respect is best described as a _____. (p. 49)
   *1.* Role
   *2.* Norm
   *3.* Value
   *4.* Commitment

**174.** A statement broadly defining the purposes and values held by a facility is a _____. (p. 50)
1. Statement of intent
2. Set of aspirations
3. Long-term goal
4. Mission statement

**175.** When the administrator concentrates on getting paperwork done, meeting regulations, and saving money, the staff _____. (p. 50)
1. Are freed to give more attention to good patient care
2. Do the same
3. Feel the facility is being successfully managed
4. Give better quality care

**176.** The area in which it is especially important for the administrator to implement a "no excuses" approach is _____. (p. 50)
1. In preventive maintenance
2. In projecting capital needs
3. Patient care
4. Staff attitudes

**177.** It is easier for staff to buy into and be motivated by a _____. (p. 50)
1. Day-to-day set of achievements to be reached
2. Well-organized administrator
3. Well-motivated administrator
4. Dream or vision

**178.** If a facility administrator can communicate a vision or dream _____. (pp. 50–51)
1. Goals are less necessary
2. Goals can be more easily set and achieved
3. Employee tenure will be maintained
4. Employees will stop focusing on pay rates

**179.** Corporate-generated goals or mission statements generally _____. (p. 51)
1. Motivate local facility workers
2. Enervate
3. Innovate
4. Have difficulty motivating local facility workers

**180.** Organizations need the leadership of the administrator because, in the final analysis, _____. (p. 51)
1. The administrator knows what is best
2. People need to be led
3. Someone has to be in charge
4. All organizational designs are imperfect

**181.** The actual behavior and functioning of an organization such as a nursing facility _____. (p. 51)
1. Closely resembles the plan
2. Is an implementation of the plan
3. Is relatively easily achieved
4. Is infinitely more complex and incomplete than the plan

**182.** The concept of delegation is permitting decisions to be made _____. (p. 52)
 *1.* With full information
 *2.* By the well qualified nurse
 *3.* At the lowest level possible
 *4.* At the middle level of management

**183.** In terms of the need for organizations to cope, the old phrase "if it ain't broke, don't fix it" needs to be changed to _____. (p. 52)
 *1.* If you fix it, it will break elsewhere
 *2.* If you fix it too often, effectiveness will be lost
 *3.* If you don't fix it all the time, it will break
 *4.* Fixing it all the time is counterproductive

## 1.6.7 ADDITIONAL RELATED CONCEPTS

**184.** How people relate to each other in the organization, the overall style or feel of an organization, is referred to as _____. (p. 52)
 *1.* Corporate meaning
 *2.* The value system
 *3.* The corporate culture
 *4.* The personnel handbook mission statement

**185.** The concept of unity of command emphasizes the importance of each person _____. (p. 53)
 *1.* Feeling like they fit in
 *2.* Remaining on the team
 *3.* Having a meaningful role in the organization
 *4.* Being accountable to one supervisor

**186.** When the board of directors gives equal authority to manage the facility to the medical director and the administrator, the board has ignored the _____ concept. (pp. 52–53)
 *1.* Short chain of command
 *2.* Utility
 *3.* Delegation
 *4.* Unity of command

**187.** The principle that there should be as few levels of management between the chief administrator and the rank and file is the _____. (p. 53)
 *1.* Short chain of command
 *2.* Intervening levels
 *3.* Effective middle levels of managers
 *4.* Maximum use of managers

**188.** When the number of interpreters through whom information must be filtered before it reaches top management is minimized, the concept of _____ has been implemented. (p. 53)
 *1.* Balance
 *2.* Span of control
 *3.* Short chain of command
 *4.* Low profile

**189.** The administrator who pays attention to the size of the various departments, centralization and decentralization, span of control, and short chain of command is paying attention to _____. (p. 53)
  *1.* Being a good manager
  *2.* Being effective
  *3.* The concept of balance
  *4.* What is occurring in the facility

**190.** The administrator who begins with the nursing assistants' ideas then moves upwards through the director of nursing's ideas and does so for each department is utilizing the concept of _____. (p. 53)
  *1.* Management information systems
  *2.* Lowest to highest
  *3.* Respect for the individual worker
  *4.* Management by objectives

**191.** In determining the need for information, sources of information, and the amount, form and frequency of information, the administrator is considering his _____. (p. 54)
  *1.* Idea sources
  *2.* Ways of organizing the facility
  *3.* Management information system
  *4.* Record-keeping measures

**192.** The administrator tells the admissions director to drop the daily reporting and to report only on days census drops below 90%. The administrator is utilizing the _____ concept. (p. 54)
  *1.* PERT/CPM
  *2.* Delegation
  *3.* Management by objectives
  *4.* Management by exception

**193.** Mapping out time estimates for the completion of each step in renovating a wing is using _____. (pp. 54–55)
  *1.* PERT/CPM
  *2.* Delegation
  *3.* Management by objectives
  *4.* Management by exception

**194.** The administrator in the chain who is achieving the best level of resident care, but not necessarily the lowest cost per patient day, can be said to be _____, although perhaps not the most efficient administrator. (p. 55)
  *1.* Most acceptable
  *2.* Effective
  *3.* Best motivated
  *4.* The best producer

**195.** Studies of top corporate administrators suggest that these persons feel they can _____. (p. 55)
  *1.* Manage best in their industry
  *2.* Train anyone to become a top manager
  *3.* Be motivators for everyone in the organization
  *4.* Manage almost anything

**196.** The administrator who focuses on the time it takes each housekeeper to clean an area and the time it takes a nurse assistant to make a bed identifies with the _____. (p. 56)
1. Necessity to conserve time
2. Necessity to be effective
3. Scientific management school
4. Human relations school

**197.** Administrators who believe that human factors exercise the most powerful influences due to worker need to participate in social groups identify with the _____ school of management theory. (p. 56)
1. Scientific
2. Practical
3. Theoretical
4. Human relations

# 1.7
# Comparing and Controlling Quality

**198.** An administrator judging the extent to which actual results of the facility's efforts achieve the outcomes proposed in the plans is _____. (p. 58)
1. Reviewing
2. Judging
3. Achievement oriented
4. Comparing

**199.** The administrator who is successfully taking the steps necessary to adjust policies and plans of action to more satisfactorily achieve stated goals is engaged in _____. (p. 58)
1. Actively managing
2. Controlling
3. Implementing
4. Conserving resources

**200.** Translating goals into clearly stated policies, identifying appropriate measures, and stating limits to deviation are some of the requirements for _____. (p. 59)
1. Improving management
2. Effective control of quality
3. Getting ahead of competitors
4. Managing for results

**201.** Getting information in a useful form to staff at appropriate levels, stating policies of actions to be taken when limits are exceeded, and taking corrective actions are some of the requirements for _____. (p. 59)
1. Improving management
2. Effective control of quality
3. Getting ahead of competitors
4. Managing for results

**202.** Setting up a system for constant renewal of quality measures, finding control measures that are functional and valued by staff, and knowing the limitations of the scope and capabilities of a system are some of the requirements for _____. (p. 59)
1. Improving management
2. Effective control of quality
3. Getting ahead of competitors
4. Managing for results

## 1.7.2 DIAGNOSING/ORGANIZATIONAL QUALITY

**203.** Physicians diagnose and treat patient illnesses; administrators diagnose and treat _____ illnesses. (p. 60)
1. Staff
2. Corporate
3. Organizational
4. Epidemic

**204.** When an administrator studies and determines what is believed to be a problem adversely affecting the nursing facility she is engaged in a study of _____. (p. 60)
1. Human nature
2. What motivates employees
3. Organizational pathology
4. Organizational attitudes

**205.** Which of the following is not a quality measure? (p. 61)
1. Percent of staff having a good feeling about patients
2. Percent of residents who need help with activities of daily living
3. Percent of residents with urinary tract infections
4. Percent of short-stay residents with pressure sores

**206.** Managers have always sought to achieve quality control in their organizations and _____. (p. 60)
1. Clear successes have been attained across the board
2. The need for such control is a subject of controversy
3. This remains an elusive aspect of managing
4. This is largely behind us as we approach the turn of the century

**207.** Assuring that all the organizational arrangements believed needed are in place puts the emphasis on _____ as a quality measure. (p. 66)
 *1.* Structure
 *2.* Process
 *3.* Outcome
 *4.* Productivity

**208.** Focusing on the results of the effort made and the measurable impacts on the patient of care given places the emphasis on _____ as a quality measure. (p. 66)
 *1.* Structure
 *2.* Process
 *3.* Outcome
 *4.* Productivity

**209.** The federal focus on the idea that a resident's abilities in activities of daily living do not diminish unless circumstances indicate it is unavoidable places the focus on _____. (p. 67)
 *1.* Structure
 *2.* Process
 *3.* Outcome measures
 *4* Productivity

**210.** Quality, argued Deming, comes from _____. (p. 67)
 *1.* Constant inspections
 *2.* A low rework rate
 *3.* Improvement in the process
 *4.* Unswerving attention

**211.** Deming observed that too often nurses and nurse aids _____. (p. 62)
 *1.* Did not really care about doing a quality job
 *2.* Did not identify with the goals of the facility
 *3.* Learned their job from workers who were never trained properly
 *4.* Learned too much in nursing and nursing assistant training

**212.** The nurse supervisor's job, according to Deming, is to _____. (p. 62)
 *1.* Lead
 *2.* Train properly
 *3.* Set standards
 *4.* Require commitment

**213.** An atmosphere, according to Deming, in which employees feel secure enough to ask questions, take positions, and admit errors is free of _____. (p. 62)
 *1.* Serious mistakes
 *2.* Arguments
 *3.* Fear
 *4.* Refusal to work

**214.** The best source of slogans or work goals, in Deming's view, is _____. (p. 62)
 *1.* Corporate leadership
 *2.* The community
 *3.* The facility
 *4.* Each individual worker

**215.** Deming would _____ (of) setting the number of beds to be made each day or the number of rooms to be cleaned or floors scrubbed. (p. 62)
1. Approve
2. Disapprove
3. Insist on
4. See as quite functional the

**216.** In Deming's view, workers are _____. (p. 62)
1. Eager to do a good job
2. In need of constant retraining
3. Uninterested in the overall goals of the business
4. Unmotivated for the most part

**217.** Evaluation by performance, merit rating, and annual review of performance, in Deming's view, _____. (p. 63)
1. Encourage workers
2. Allow workers to know where they stand
3. Are regarded by workers as fair and needed
4. Destroy teamwork and nurture rivalry

**218.** If the administrator tells his director of nursing to compare how the facility's nursing services are organized with what he considers the best organized nursing services in the area, the administrator is _____. (p. 63)
1. Comparing
2. Contrasting
3. Benchmarking
4. Trying to improve

**219.** A benchmarking effort _____ be justified by seeking out significantly better practices rather than solely focusing on best practices. (p. 64)
1. Can rarely
2. Can
3. Never is
4. Always can

**220.** When Deming warned not to simply copy others' efforts when benchmarking, he was advocating _____. (p. 65)
1. A new approach to benchmarking
2. Less benchmarking
3. Improved benchmarking
4. Adapting, rather than copying benchmarked ideas

**221.** Total organizational involvement in improving all aspects of quality of service is the goal of _____. (p. 65)
1. Total quality management
2. New management
3. Spectrum management
4. Management by objective

**222.** The approach in total quality of management of placing responsibility with the workers who produce a service is sometimes known as _____. (p. 65)
1. Source management
2. Outsourcing
3. Quality at the source
4. Worker involvement

**223.** Employee empowerment in decision making, use of teams, and use of individual responsibility for services characterizes _____. (p. 65)
1. Management by quality
2. Resource maximization
3. Total quality management
4. Benchmarking

**224.** In the American Hospital Association's view, the goal of total quality management is to _____ customer expectations. (pp. 65–66)
1. Meet
2. Anticipate
3. Exceed
4. Analyze

**225.** Visionary CEOs acting as coaches, commitment to customers, and trained teams characterize _____. (pp. 65–66)
1. Successful benchmarking
2. The Deming analysis and recommendation
3. Total quality management
4. Management by objectives

**226.** Experience suggests that successful total quality management can be implemented in an organization over a period of _____. (pp. 65–66)
1. 5 to 10 months
2. 5 to 10 years
3. 2 to 3 years
4. Under 1 year if the organization is fully committed

**227.** Managing for quality consists of quality planning, quality control, and _____. (pp. 65–66)
1. Knowing the difference
2. Being able to see the difference
3. Quality improvement
4. Benchmarking

# 1.8
# Innovating

**228.** Bringing new ideas into the way an organization accomplishes its purposes is the result of _____. (p. 73)
1. Hard work
2. Predicting the future
3. Innovating
4. Quality improvement

**229.** The role of innovator is _____. (p. 73)
1. Best assigned to the administrator
2. Available to all employees
3. A skill employees are able to develop
4. Best taught in inservices

**230.** One writer suggests that managers should _____ specific objectives that will guide the organization over an extended period of time. (p. 74)
1. Avoid trying to set out too
2. Encourage
3. Assign
4. Insist on

**231.** In the nursing facility, innovation is _____. (p. 74)
1. Seldom encountered
2. The prerogative of middle and upper management
3. Finding new solutions to creating quality of life for residents
4. An ever elusive goal

**232.** Innovation can be expected _____. (pp. 73–75)
1. From all levels in a nursing home chain
2. Primarily from upper-level management
3. Primarily from ownership
4. From middle-level well trained staff who have the opportunity to update their skills

# 1.9
# Marketing the Long-term Care Facility

## 1.9.1 THE TURN TO MARKETING

**233.** Like many hospitals, nursing homes are increasingly turning to _____ to maintain satisfactory income. (p. 76)
1. Corporate bonds
2. Filling a market niche
3. Stock offerings
4. Increasing the profit margins achieved

**234.** When a facility has achieved the premier status as the best caregiver in the community, experience suggests that it will likely _____. (p. 76)
1. Retain that position over time
2. Lull itself into complacency
3. Make an even greater effort to retain its position
4. Seek additional ways to maintain that position

**235.** In today's competitive market, good nursing facilities _____. (p. 76)
1. Abound
2. Are scarce
3. Seldom are identifiable
4. Have disappeared

**236.** The downside of being a good nursing facility is that it _____. (p. 76)
1. Causes staff to stop trying
2. Is difficult to maintain
3. Is not recognized by the public
4. Only puts you with the rest of the pack

## 1.9.2 THE "MARKETING" OF HEALTH CARE

**237.** Several years ago the U.S. Supreme Court _____ self-imposed restrictions by health and other professionals against advertising services or prices that have the result of keeping the public ignorant or inhibiting free flow of information. (p. 77)
1. Ruled as permissible
2. Discouraged, but did not rule illegal
3. Ruled illegal
4. Permitted

**238.** Competition occurs when two or more organizations seek to serve _____ in an exchange process. (p. 77)
1. Two or more groups
2. Four or more groups
3. Numerous individuals
4. The same individual or group

**239.** The audit, market segmentation, choosing a market mix, implementing the plan, evaluation of results, and control are the steps in _____. (p. 78)
1. Managing by objectives
2. Total quality management
3. Marketing
4. Good management

**240.** The marketing of the nursing facility is in a special context because of _____. (pp. 78–79)
1. Special laws covering nursing facility marketing
2. Public ambivalence toward the nursing facility
3. Special costs to the nursing facility not borne by other providers
4. Restrictive legislation governing nursing facility marketing practices

## 1.9.3 DEVELOPING A MARKETING STRATEGY

**241.** Selecting a target market or markets, choosing a competitive position, and developing an effective marketing mix to reach and serve the identified customers is _____. (p. 79)
1. Unnecessary for the typical nursing facility
2. Necessary only in states where no certificate of need exists
3. Developing a marketing strategy
4. Implementing good planning and directing

**242.** A marketing strategy includes _____. (p. 79)
1. Excessive sums of money
2. Hiring an outside firm
3. Hiring a marketing person
4. Selecting a target

**243.** The administrator asks a committee to engage in the process of identifying, collecting, and analyzing information about the external environment. In marketing terminology the administrator is seeking a/an _____. (p. 81)
1. Environmental analysis
2. Audit
3. Segmented market
4. Multiple market

**244.** The percent of residents whose selected medical conditions were being treated as a medical condition requiring special care is _____. (p. 80)
1. Ostomy care
2. Radiation therapy
3. Tube feeding
4. Mechanically altered diets

**245.** When the administrator decides to serve only longer-term residents, Medicare residents, and Alzheimer's residents, in marketing terminology, the administrator has selected the _____. (p. 81)
1. Product mix
2. Targets
3. Goals
4. Opportunities

**246.** The percent of residents whose health condition is being treated as a medical condition requiring special care in rehabilitation is _____. (p. 81)
1. 2
2. 20
3. 70
4. 91

**247.** The steps of problem recognition, information search, alternative evaluation, purchase decision, and post-purchase evaluation are, in marketing texts, identified as the steps in _____. (p. 83)
1. Consumer decision making
2. Facility market segmentation decisions
3. Health care marketing practices
4. Government rule making

**248.** Factors such as general appearance of the facility, absence of odors, and the appearance of the patients may be factors of which the decision maker may not be consciously aware in visiting a facility into which to place a relative. These are referred to as _____ factors. (p. 84)
1. Key
2. Special
3. Usual
4. Subliminal

**249.** Normally, one of the most effective marketing tools is _____. (p. 84)
1. Advertising
2. Staff recommendations
3. A tour through the facility
4. Hiring a consultant

**250.** Cognitive readiness, affective readiness, and behavioral readiness are _____. (p. 85)
1. A complex marketing theory
2. The steps in marketing
3. The goals of advertising
4. Often not cost effective

# NAB Domain: Human Resources

# Understanding the Departments and Managing Human Resources

## 2.1

# Organizational Patterning of the Nursing Facility and Its Staff

**1.** One practical reason the administrator must rely more and more on the expertise of department heads is _____. (p. 91)
   1. Requirements are too numerous for one person to remember
   2. Department heads are being better trained
   3. Department heads are coming with more experience
   4. Department heads care more

**2.** One overarching consideration in deciding at what level, that is, the number of nursing hours per patient day, to staff the facility is _____. (p. 91)
   1. Ownership needs
   2. Medical complexity of care given
   3. Number of patients
   4. State and federal minimum staffing requirements

**3.** The one person most responsible for resident rights in the nursing facility is the _____. (p. 94)
   1. Administrator
   2. Direct caregiver
   3. Director of nursing
   4. Resident council president

**4.** Quality assessment and control, infection control, and physical plant health and safety are _____. (p. 93)
1. New requirements
2. Long-standing requirements
3. Federally required committees
4. Federally required committees and/or functions

**5.** Generally, the percentage of nursing facilities with deficiencies for resident rights in 2008 was _____. (p. 96)
1. Over 15
2. Unacceptable
3. Under 3
4. Under 15

**6.** In the typical nursing facility of 100 patients, the administrator normally has _____ reporting to her. (pp. 92–93)
1. 17 department heads
2. 6 middle-level managers
3. 7 or 8 department heads
4. 3 or 4 department heads

**7.** Larger facilities (of 200 or more patients) might consider the appointment of perhaps _____ middle-level managers to whom two or more department heads may report. (p. 92)
1. Two
2. Three
3. Four
4. Half a dozen

**8.** Activities such as assuring quality of care for all residents, advocating for all residents, and developing and managing the budget are normally associated most closely with the _____. (p. 94)
1. Business office
2. Admissions team
3. Nursing area
4. Administrator's office

**9.** In 2008, U.S. nursing facilities achieved _____ compliance with physician services. (pp. 95–97)
1. 50%
2. 60%
3. 75%
4. 98% or more

**10.** Activities such as empowering department heads, setting the tone, and settling territorial disputes are normally associated most closely with the _____. (p. 94)
1. Business office
2. Admissions team
3. Nursing area
4. Administrator's office

**11.** The rate of compliance with dental requirements in U.S. facilities in 2008 was _____.
(p. 99)
*1.* Less than 50%
*2.* 80%
*3.* 99%
*4.* 100%

**12.** Federal congressionally written requirements for the role(s) the medical director
may/must play are _____. (p. 97)
*1.* Brief and vague
*2.* Detailed and extensive
*3.* Constantly changing
*4.* Becoming increasingly burdensome in recent years

**13.** When attending physicians fail to visit their patients on a timely basis the medical
director _____. (p. 95)
*1.* Often substitutes and accomplishes the required physician services
*2.* Never substitutes
*3.* Must send federally required reminders notices
*4.* Must provide mandatory counseling with these physicians

**14.** In most nursing facilities of 100 to 120 beds, there is _____ medical staff. (p. 95)
*1.* Always an organized
*2.* Usually no organized
*3.* An open
*4.* A closed

**15.** Pharmacy services in U.S. nursing facilities in 2008 were about 98% in compliance
with the exception of _____. (p. 100)
*1.* Procedures and storage
*2.* Drug passes
*3.* Record keeping
*4.* Giving medications on a timely basis

**16.** One of the main advantages of a closed medical staff is that _____. (pp. 95–96)
*1.* One of them can be on call all the time
*2.* Cost savings are realized
*3.* Patients are more satisfied with the care given
*4.* Patients like the broader choice available

**17.** Facility compliance with laboratory services requirements in 2008 was _____.
(p. 101)
*1.* Less than earlier
*2.* The basis for closing several facilities
*3.* About 75%
*4.* Nearly 100%

**18.** Closed medical staffs are more likely in _____ facilities that serve a large _____ patient population. (pp. 96–97)
   *1.* Smaller/Medicare
   *2.* Medium sized/Medicare
   *3.* Larger/Medicare
   *4.* Larger/Medicaid

**19.** Dental care is often a neglected area of care in nursing facilities because dentists _____. (pp. 97–98)
   *1.* Are typically reimbursed approximately half the office fee
   *2.* Are not interested in the geriatric population
   *3.* Feel less care is needed in the geriatric population
   *4.* Are not trained to care for older persons

**20.** Dental care is also often a neglected area of care in nursing facilities because dentists _____. (pp. 97–98)
   *1.* Are often insecure about functioning outside their office with complex cases
   *2.* Are not eligible for Medicare reimbursement
   *3.* Are not eligible for Medicaid reimbursement
   *4.* Are nearly all overworked and have no time available

**21.** Total RN and LPN hours per patient day in U.S. nursing facilities during 1993–2005 _____. (pp. 102–103)
   *1.* Remained unchanged
   *2.* Rose perceptibly then decreased slightly
   *3.* Decreased
   *4.* Reflected the nursing shortage

**22.** Successful solutions to oral care in the facility will likely be linked to _____. (pp. 97–98)
   *1.* Training a local dentist
   *2.* Paying a higher-than-office rate
   *3.* Retaining a dental director at perhaps $2.00 to $4.00 per patient per month
   *4.* Arranging for care through the local dental school

**23.** There is need in most nursing facilities for a _____ who will make rounds seeing patients on a monthly basis and train nursing staff to observe and meet patients' oral needs. (p. 98)
   *1.* Dental technician
   *2.* Dentist
   *3.* Dental assistant
   *4.* Dental hygienist

**24.** One practical solution to attaining a satisfactory level of oral care for nursing facility patients is to _____. (p. 98)
   *1.* Contract with several dentists for weekly visits
   *2.* Hire two or three dental hygienists
   *3.* Train oral care aides (a regularly employed nurses aide)
   *4.* Seek Medicaid reimbursement for oral care given

**25.** A podiatrist is an important component of foot care in the nursing facility because
_____. (pp. 98–99)
1. People like good care of their feet
2. Residents walk a lot
3. Diabetics need podiatrists for safe toenail clipping
4. Medicaid requires it on a monthly basis

**26.** Assuring all medications are available as ordered, that all reorders and stop orders
are implemented, and reviewing each patient's medications monthly falls to the
_____. (p. 99)
1. Local pharmacy
2. Pharmacists providing medications to the facility
3. Director of nurses
4. Consulting pharmacist

**27.** Observing medication passes and recording and reporting drug error rates falls to
the _____. (p. 99)
1. Director of nursing
2. Consulting pharmacist
3. Administrator's office
4. Medical director

**28.** A facility of 120 patients with eight new admission per month might _____ physical
therapy services. (pp. 100–101)
1. Contract for
2. Provide in-house
3. Routinely send residents out for
4. Not offer

**29.** A facility of 120 patients with 30–40 new admissions each month will likely _____
physical therapy services. (pp. 100–101)
1. Offer in-house
2. Contract for a few hours per week any
3. Not offer
4. Routinely send residents out for

**30.** One way some facilities have bridged the gap between formal physical therapy given
and the "habilitative" care given daily by the nursing staff is to _____. (p. 100)
1. Place a physical therapist on staff
2. Use an occupational therapist in addition
3. Train all nurses in physical therapy
4. Establish a restorative nursing program led by a nurse

**31.** Increasingly, facilities needing X-rays are _____. (p. 101)
1. Calling 911
2. Using local buses for the handicapped
3. Using mobile X-ray services
4. Installing their own X-ray department with staff

**32.** In the nursing facility, implanted ports, mid-line catheters, central line catheters, and epidural lines are part of _____. (p. 103)
1. Routine nursing
2. Intensive care unit nursing
3. Subacute care
4. New wave health care

**33.** For nursing to achieve its tasks, _____. (p. 103)
1. Nearly every department must cooperate
2. Well-trained staff are desirable
3. Inservices must be routine
4. Nurses must care deeply

**34.** Keeping medical records must be assigned to _____. (p. 108)
1. A part-time employee
2. A well-trained employee
3. A medical records specialist
4. A full-time employee

**35.** The major difference between the challenge facing the nursing home dietary director compared to the hospital dietary director is _____. (p. 108)
1. Fewer patients to feed
2. Less staff
3. Diets over an extended period of time
4. Patient preferences

**36.** During the years 1993–2008, the major area in dietary services that needed improvement in the view of the inspectors was _____. (p. 110)
1. Taste of the food
2. Sanitary conditions
3. Presentation of food
4. Feeding styles

**37.** A particular patient-care-related concern the administrator should address when evaluating the social worker and activities director's work is _____. (p. 113)
1. Whether they are well trained
2. Whether they like their jobs
3. Whether less responsive patients are receiving attention
4. How well they interact with other staff

**38.** Deficiencies for housekeeping appear to be _____. (pp. 119–120)
1. Varying over time
2. Going up
3. Degrading
4. Fully acceptable

## 2.2
# Identifying the Human Resources Functions

**39.** The personnel for which the personnel director has line responsibility is _____. (p. 123)
1. All staff
2. Staff outside of the nursing area
3. Personnel department staff
4. New-hires still in the 90-day initial employment period

**40.** In practice, most of the actual hiring in nursing facilities is done by the _____. (p. 123)
1. Director of personnel
2. Director of nursing
3. Administrator
4. Department managers

**41.** In the typical facility of 100 patients there is/are _____ full-time personnel director(s). (p. 123)
1. One
2. Two
3. No
4. A professionally trained

## 2.3
# Planning Employment Needs: Writing Job Descriptions

**42.** The process of defining a job in terms of tasks or behaviors required and specifying the qualifications is performing a _____. (p. 125)
1. Job specification
2. Job description
3. Job analysis
4. Job evaluation

**43.** Information about the job that results in a statement of the job to be done, including a list of duties, title, and qualifications is a job _____. (p. 125)
   *1.* Specification
   *2.* Description
   *3.* Analysis
   *4.* Evaluation

**44.** That which distinguishes one job from all others is the job _____. (p. 125)
   *1.* Specification
   *2.* Description
   *3.* Title
   *4.* Evaluation

**45.** A coordinated and aggregated series of work elements used to produce an output, for example, making a bed, is known as a _____. (p. 125)
   *1.* Job specification
   *2.* Job description
   *3.* Task
   *4.* Job evaluation

**46.** The administrator asks the financial manager to identify competition for personnel, estimate in-migration or out-migration of workers, and look at wage scales in the area. The administrator wants _____. (p. 127)
   *1.* An orientation to the area
   *2.* A job family to be established
   *3.* A person power inventory
   *4.* More information than is needed

**47.** The authority of government agencies to review facility recruitment sources, advertising and statistics on the number of applicants, and persons hired by category stems from _____. (p. 128)
   *1.* The Americans with Disabilities Act
   *2.* The Equal Opportunities Commission
   *3.* The Civil Rights Act
   *4.* New federal powers

**48.** The geographical scope of a search for applicants for a nursing assistant or housekeeping job is likely to be limited to _____. (p. 129)
   *1.* The state
   *2.* Commuting distance
   *3.* The county
   *4.* That region of the United States

**49.** Present employees, career ladders, job-posting, and job-bidding are _____. (pp. 129–130)
   *1.* Inappropriate recruiting sources
   *2.* Good recruiting sources
   *3.* Too expensive as recruiting sources
   *4.* Unrelated to the applicant pool

**50.** Career ladders are paths along which the employee (p. 129)
   1. Finds limitations
   2. Is restricted
   3. Finds unlimited options
   4. Can hope to progress

**51.** Posting a job opening on the facility bulletin board is _____. (p. 129)
   1. Generally a good practice
   2. Required by the EEOC
   3. Required by the Civil Rights Act
   4. Poor personnel practice

**52.** Use of a search firm would be more appropriate for hiring a _____. (p. 131)
   1. New director of activities
   2. Well-qualified nurse
   3. New administrator
   4. Registered dietitian

# 2.6
# Hiring Staff

**53.** Recruitment is the process of _____ prospective staff. (p. 133)
   1. Locating
   2. Screening
   3. Interviewing
   4. Placing

**54.** Personnel selection is the process of _____. (p. 133)
   1. Deciding which applicant best fits the job requirements
   2. Setting up interviews with applicants
   3. Reviewing interview results
   4. Hiring and firing

**55.** Prohibiting discrimination on the basis of race, color, religion, sex, or national origin is the basis of the _____. (p. 133)
   1. Wagner Act
   2. Civil Legislation Act
   3. Employment Act
   4. Civil Rights Act

**56.** The Civil Rights Act Title 7 and the Equal Employment Act of 1972 apply to employers of _____ or more employees. (p. 133)
1. 50
2. 100
3. 200
4. 15

**57.** The employer interviews 90 Black applicants and 30 white applicants, then hires 30 white and 30 Black applicants. If applicants were hired in these proportions over time, the facility would likely experience _____. (p. 133)
1. Reverse impact
2. Reverse discrimination
3. Worker pool depletion
4. Adverse impact

**58.** The staff development coordinator sent a candidate to five different department heads who used her newly developed application form and obtained the same score results. The staff development coordinator can reasonably feel her application form has _____. (p. 136)
1. Reasonable reliability
2. Good validity
3. A great future
4. Construct validity

**59.** The staff development coordinator asks several of the department heads if the application form she has developed is helping them match candidates with job descriptions. She is wondering if the instrument has _____. (p. 136)
1. Content validity
2. Reliability
3. Usefulness
4. Repeatability

**60.** The staff development coordinator has found an instrument that measures a trait believed important to jobs in nursing facilities. The staff development coordinator believes this instrument has _____. (p. 135)
1. Construct validity
2. Reliability
3. Definite usefulness
4. Content validity

**61.** The director of nurses asks an applicant for her age and religious affiliation. This is _____. (p. 137)
1. Illegal
2. Encouraged
3. Necessary to the interview
4. Permissible under certain circumstances

**62.** After hiring an applicant, the staff development coordinator demands that the new hire bring in a photograph or allow one to be made at the facility. This is _____. (p. 137)
1. Illegal
2. Legal
3. Necessary to the interview
4. Permissible under certain circumstances

**63.** The director of nurses asks the applicant nurse if he is willing to work Easter. This is _____. (p. 136)
1. Illegal
2. Legal
3. Necessary to the interview
4. Permissible under certain circumstances

**64.** The director of nurses asks the nurse candidate how much alcohol she consumes per week. This is _____. (p. 136)
1. Illegal
2. Legal
3. Necessary to the interview
4. Permissible under certain circumstances

**65.** The director of nurses asks the applicant whether he has ever been treated for drug problems. This is _____. (p. 136)
1. Illegal
2. Legal
3. Necessary to the interview
4. Permissible under certain circumstances

**66.** The director of nursing asks the treatment nurse applicant a predetermined and set array of questions. The director of nursing is using a/an _____ interview approach. (p. 139)
1. Nondirective
2. Directive
3. In-depth
4. Patterned

**67.** A director of nursing asking a nurse supervisor applicant, "What actions have you taken if you disagreed with a supervisor's decision?" is _____. (p. 140)
1. Illegal
2. Legal
3. Necessary to the interview
4. Permissible under certain circumstances

**68.** Research results suggest that interviews for job applicants may be better for explaining _____. (p. 140)
1. Why a person would not be a good candidate
2. Why a person is a good candidate
3. What truly motivates the applicant
4. The applicant's true value system

69. When asked, an applicant reveals she has been convicted in an area relevant to the job being sought. The director of nursing then considers the nature, number, facts surrounding, job-relatedness, and length of time since or between convictions. This is _____. (p. 141)
    1. Illegal
    2. Legal
    3. Necessary to the interview
    4. Permissible under certain circumstances

70. Credit reports on job applicants _____. (p. 142)
    1. Require the applicant's permission
    2. Are routinely done
    3. Are usually not meaningful
    4. Are illegal

71. A good risk-management-related reason for requiring a physical exam before any new employee begins work is to _____. (p. 142)
    1. Discover any handicaps
    2. Be able to assess the employee's future health needs
    3. Be able to inform relevant staff of any limitations
    4. Provide a baseline against which to assess later exams or claims

72. If the physician determines the new employee cannot perform essential functions of the position accepted due to a disability covered under the Americans With Disabilities Act, the facility _____. (p. 142)
    1. Must assist in finding placement in another facility
    2. Must make a reasonable accommodation
    3. Inform the applicant of his unsuitability
    4. Put the new hire to work on the position hired for

73. In most nursing facilities, the final decision to hire a job applicant is made by the _____. (p. 144)
    1. Director of personnel
    2. Staff development coordinator
    3. Administrator
    4. Department head

74. Thirty years ago, successful caring for the frail elderly in the facility often depended less on technical knowledge than compassion for others. Today, successful caring for the frail elderly in the facility increasingly depends on _____. (p. 144)
    1. Technical knowledge
    2. Even more compassion
    3. Both technical knowledge and compassion
    4. Ability to perform the job specifications

**75.** Nurses and nursing assistants who have drive and enthusiasm for caring for the patient _____. (p. 145)
1. Have everything necessary
2. Have the essential ingredients
3. Can be taught technical skills they lack
4. Have a reduced role in the modern facility

**76.** Applicants who lack fire in their hearts or passion for their work _____. (p. 145)
1. Are relatively easy to fire up
2. Are not so easily taught
3. Need to be technically competent to compensate
4. Are still good candidates if technically competent

**77.** The hiring decision itself _____. (p. 145)
1. Is complex
2. Takes care of itself
3. Is usually clear
4. Should be done based on numbers

# 2.7
# Training Staff

**78.** The first day on the job _____. (p. 146)
1. Is usually a blur
2. Is less important than later
3. Leaves a lasting impression
4. Produces little output

**79.** Official welcome, introduction to staff, and tour of facility are activities best associated with the _____. (p. 146)
1. First week on the job
2. Pre-job visit
3. First day on the job
4. Orientation, at some point

**80.** Valuable tax credits can be achieved if the facility assures employees comply with the _____. (p. 147)
1. Civil Rights Acts requirements
2. Americans With Disabilities Act
3. Tax credit for handicapped workers
4. Targeted Jobs Tax Credit Program

**81.** A compilation of facility policies that directly relate to work conditions is _____. (p. 147)
1. The employee contract
2. The pre-employment orientation
3. A legal agreement between employer and employee
4. The employee handbook

**82.** Employers who have entered clear disclaimers in the employee handbook have _____ successful employee suits in court, alleging the handbook to be a binding contract. (p. 147)
1. Prevented
2. Encouraged
3. Proliferated
4. Not prevented

**83.** When the staff development coordinator reviews job descriptions and the activities essential for performing each job, he is performing a _____. (p. 148)
1. Service to the facility
2. Needed personnel action
3. Task analysis
4. Employee skill analysis

**84.** Employee education offered throughout the work career of the employee, often of a mandatory nature, is typically referred to as _____. (p. 149)
1. Skill sharpening
2. Continuing education
3. Seminars
4. Inservices

**85.** One way to improve evaluation of training efforts is to state learning objectives _____. (p. 150)
1. As learning objectives
2. As objectively as possible
3. In quantifiable terms
4. As behavioral objectives

# 2.8

# Retaining Employees

**86.** Social approval, self-esteem, security, and use of power are examples of (what) _____. (p. 151)
1. Employers seek from employees
2. Each employer offers employees
3. Employees seek from the facility
4. Overly idealistic goals

87. Generally, if the community or significant others disapprove of the employee working at a facility, the employee _____. (p. 152)
    1. Will quit
    2. Will redouble her effort
    3. Not have positive feelings about working at the facility
    4. Will be enabled by facility attitude to ignore this

88. Being part of a facility that has a sense of purpose to which an employee can dedicate energy with pride enhances an employee's _____. (p. 152)
    1. Merit pay expectations
    2. Sense of destiny
    3. Willingness to volunteer
    4. Self-esteem

89. Employees who are enjoying a high level of job satisfaction are more likely to be able to _____. (p. 153)
    1. Require additional benefits
    2. Have been to significant inservice training sessions
    3. Achieve educational goals
    4. Provide a high level of patient care

90. Employees want to work for an employer that _____. (p. 152)
    1. Pays outstanding stock dividends
    2. Has an AAA rating in the market
    3. Has a great education program
    4. Stimulates their dreams and aspirations

91. Among the following, the staff most need the administrator to _____. (p. 152)
    1. Provide a large array of educational options
    2. Assure that the bonuses are distributed equitably
    3. Meet their self-actuating needs
    4. Take a personal interest in them

92. Every day, administrators in more than 16,000 nursing facilities make personnel decisions based on _____. (p. 153)
    1. What they were taught in personnel class
    2. The psychologist they most admire
    3. The theories they have read and assimilated
    4. Their assumptions of what motivates the staff

93. The assumptions that employees naturally dislike work, prefer to receive extensive direction from superiors, and work to avoid responsibility characterized the _____. (p. 153)
    1. Human relations school
    2. Scientific management school
    3. Theory X philosophy
    4. Theory Y philosophy

**94.** Managers who believe that using energy to work is as natural as using energy to play or rest, that individuals can exercise self-direction, and both seek and accept responsibility accept the approach characterized as the _____. (p. 153)
   1. Human relations school
   2. Scientific management school
   3. Theory X philosophy
   4. Theory Y philosophy

**95.** A test often used by facility personnel staff that has 100 questions asking respondents how they feel or act in a variety of situations, then places respondents into categories of introverted or extroverted, sensing or intuitive, thinking or feeling, and perceiving or judging is the _____. (p. 154)
   1. Complete Personality Analyses Series
   2. Myers-Briggs Type Indicator
   3. Left-brain, right-brain analysis
   4. Simpsons Personality Series

**96.** Persons characterized as systematic, thorough, and balanced and who ask detailed questions about each situation are characterized as _____. (p. 154)
   1. Right brained
   2. Left brained
   3. Influenced
   4. Balanced

**97.** Persons characterized as more intuitive, quick, and less complex in their approach to decision making are characterized as (p. 154)
   1. Right brained
   2. Left brained
   3. Influenced
   4. Balanced

**98.** One safer generalization about employee motives is that _____. (p. 155)
   1. They are predictable
   2. They are always mixed
   3. Little is known about them
   4. They are manageable

**99.** Some motives/needs may recede when satisfied, for example, hunger or thirst; other motives such as the need for power _____. (p. 155)
   1. Follow the same pattern
   2. Are unpredictable
   3. Disappear when met
   4. May become more intensified when partially achieved

**100.** The process of giving employees increased roles in the decision making processes of the facility is sometimes called _____. (p. 155)
   1. Overuse of resources
   2. Under use of management authority and direction
   3. Division of power
   4. Job enrichment

**101.** In Maslow's hierarchy of needs concept, it is _____ to meet lower needs before higher needs become salient. (p. 156)
1. Necessary
2. Easy
3. Incorrect
4. Optional

**102.** Employees who are hard-driving and achievement-oriented, who strive constantly to achieve higher levels are characterized as _____. (p. 156)
1. Type A
2. Type B
3. Driven
4. Successful

**103.** Persons who have only moderate achievement needs, are less competitive, and more satisfied with moderation whether in sports, titles, or on-the-job productivity are characterized as _____. (p. 156)
1. Type A
2. Type B
3. Less driven
4. Cool

**104.** A concept or idea that supplies enthusiasm, vigor, and direction to the facility's efforts is referred to by Kriegel as a _____. (p. 158)
1. Supreme motivator
2. Dream or vision
3. Finest alternative
4. Best motivator

**105.** Short-term targets to be achieved, such as assuring that all the paperwork is done for new admissions in a timely manner, are referred to by Kriegel as _____. (p. 158)
1. Supremely motivating
2. A dream or vision
3. Goals
4. Best motivators

**106.** A charge nurse being encouraged to become a nurse practitioner, and a nurses aide being supported to become a licensed practical nurse are examples of a facility commitment to provide employees _____. (p. 158)
1. A good chance to get ahead
2. Upward mobility
3. More education
4. A career path

**107.** In Kriegel's view, failure is a good place to start; the major downside to failure occurring is when the employee ____. (p. 159)
1. Feels bad about the failure
2. Gets it right the next time
3. Does not cause real harm
4. Fails to learn from failure

**108.** The facility administration's attitude toward error, argues Kriegel, is critical to success. In his view, mistakes _____. (p. 159)
1. Can be minimized
2. Ought to be intercepted early
3. Must be interpreted
4. Are inevitable and are an opportunity to learn

**109.** Employees prefer to work in a facility in which mistakes _____. (p. 159)
1. Are not emphasized
2. Are forgiven
3. Are expected
4. Are kept from harming anyone

**110.** The medication nurse who bursts into the director of nurses' office and bemoans making a 20% error rate on her last attempt to pass medications has _____. (p. 159)
1. Put the facility into jeopardy
2. Failed to do reasonable risk management
3. Really messed up
4. Set the stage for communication and improvement

**111.** The idea that when reward follows performance, performance improves and that when rewards do not follow performance, performance deteriorates is known as _____. (p. 159)
1. Expectancy theory
2. Reward theory
3. Reinforcement theory
4. A flawed approach

**112.** The reduction in degrees of freedom in decision making brought about by well-developed policies is _____. (p. 160)
1. Always a plus
2. The crux of a good risk-management program
3. A potential downside of having good policies
4. The conformity it is necessary to assure

**113.** Department heads who conform, are defensive, produce detailed substantiation of unimportant problems, and give invalid information illustrate _____. (p. 160)
1. Argyris's belief that organizations tend to treat employees as immature
2. That organizations need good communication channels
3. Today's organizations
4. How they may actually be helping the organization

**114.** The idea of treating each employee as a member of the team is _____. (p. 161)
1. An unrealistic goal
2. Not functional in a nursing facility setting
3. An effort to combat powerlessness, to give employees "ownership"
4. Always effective

**115.** A director of nursing consulting aides on whether they are prepared to receive a new admission and acting on the aides' decision is an attempt to _____. (p. 161)
1. Give ownership to the aides, and treat them as "businesspersons"
2. Be sensitive to the aides' work loads
3. Get advice from all sources
4. Be a good communicator

**116.** One of the major tasks of the administrator is to _____. (p. 162)
1. Treat employees civilly
2. Be supportive of employees needs
3. Create and enforce opportunities for staff to feel in control
4. Create opportunities for staff to vent their feelings

**117.** High patient care depends, in part, on whether the administrator is able to _____. (p. 162)
1. Reward staff sufficiently
2. Defend staff to residents and families
3. Create career ladders for all staff
4. Enable the employees to "buy" into the facility

**118.** "It'll never work, we've tried that 20 times already," "yeah, but…" are common responses to new suggestions known as _____. (pp. 162–163)
1. Negation
2. Not invented here
3. Circular nature of organizations
4. Fire hoses

**119.** In Kriegel's view, there are immense pressures in the contemporary world leading to a faster is better mentality. His view is that _____. (p. 163)
1. This is inevitable
2. This can be mitigated slightly
3. One should go with the flow
4. Creativity and innovation are losers to speed

**120.** In Kriegel's view, the 100% effort required when "we're working short today" leads to _____. He prefers a _____. (p. 164)
1. Job dissatisfaction/passionate 90%
2. Needed staffing reviews/100% effort
3. Frustration/70% effort
4. Use of pool personnel/use of regular staff

**121.** Aristotle is said to have observed that pleasure in the job puts perfection in the work. To Kriegel this means the facility should _____. (p. 164)
1. Appoint Ninjas of joy
2. Increase the activities substantially
3. Hire fun-loving staff
4. Seek pleasure, whatever the cost

# 2.9
# Evaluating Employees

122. There are those, such as Deming, who argue that being the member of a productive team affords the facility managers sufficient evaluation and control over employees' performance. One potential problem with this is that _____. (p. 165)
    1. It fosters team membership
    2. It stifles creativity
    3. Organizations' memories are short
    4. Employees like to have written records of their work

123. Job performance evaluation is intended to be a function of comparing and controlling personnel _____. (p. 166)
    1. Attitudes
    2. Approaches to management
    3. Behavior
    4. Performance quality

124. The absence of any written system for evaluation of long-term performance exposes the individual more nearly to _____. (p. 166)
    1. Good judgment of current managers
    2. Evaluation on present work
    3. Higher appraisals
    4. The whim of managers

125. Employees, it has been observed, normally _____. (p. 166)
    1. Outperform their self-image
    2. Do not outperform their self-image
    3. Are self-starting, for the most part
    4. Require little supervision in the traditional nursing facility setting

126. An evaluator checking off the extent to which an employee meets a trait or requirement is using a/an _____. (p. 167)
    1. Outmoded model
    2. Performance scale
    3. Rating scale
    4. Global rating

127. Department heads who consistently give high ratings to avoid conflict illustrate the _____. (p. 168)
    1. Abuse of global ratings
    2. Leniency error
    3. Error of central tendency
    4. Halo effect

**128.** The supervisor is impressed by the fact that the employee never missed a day and was never late, so rated the employee highly overall. This is a/an_____. (p. 168)
   1. Abuse of global ratings
   2. Leniency error
   3. Error of central tendency
   4. Halo effect

**129.** Transfer, promotion, demotion, and layoff are possible outcomes of _____. (p. 168)
   1. Poor work attitudes
   2. A performance appraisal
   3. Good rating scales at work
   4. Global ratings for some managers

# 2.10
# Paying Employees

**130.** Workers expecting an exchange in which their wages and benefits are equal to their work effort when compared to similarly situated employees illustrate the _____. (p. 171)
   1. Resiliency of worker expectation
   2. Fair exchange theory
   3. Compensation theory
   4. Equity theory

**131.** Giving an across-the-board wage increase based on the Consumer Price Index is giving a/an _____. (p. 172)
   1. Well-deserved raise to the staff
   2. Boost in staff pay levels
   3. Cost of living increase
   4. Indexed wage increase

**132.** In the nursing facility, the key job against which many staff measure their wages is compensation of the _____. (p. 172)
   1. Administrator
   2. Medical director
   3. Owner
   4. Director of nursing

# 2.11
# Disciplining Employees

**133.** Unless the facility can convincingly illustrate that it had a "just cause" for firing an employee, that employee will likely _____. (p. 174)
1. Be rehired
2. Remain on the facility payroll
3. Collect unemployment
4. Complain to the state

**134.** Grievance procedures offer a needed _____. (p. 174)
1. Source of discipline
2. Safety valve
3. Protection to the management
4. Reciprocity relationship

# 3

## NAB Domain: Finance/Business

# Learning to Manage the Organization's Finances

1. The staff person responsible for assuring that the business office runs smoothly is, in the final analysis, _____. (p. 179)
   1. Corporate finance director
   2. The administrator
   3. Business office staff
   4. Facility treasurer

2. In general, the ownership patterns for U.S. nursing facilities in 2008 _____. (p. 180)
   1. Was consistent with 1993 and 1999
   2. Were changing rapidly
   3. Varied widely from state to state
   4. Were unchanged from three decades earlier

3. Generating reports on the financial standing of the nursing facility is generally assigned to _____. (p. 179)
   1. The accountant
   2. The director of financial
   3. The administrative assistant
   4. The chief financial officer (CFO)

4. Responsibility and blame for overspending in the department of nursing and in food services is typically assigned by the owners to the _____. (p. 180)
   1. Director of nursing and director of food services
   2. Director of nursing and the dietitian
   3. Chief financial officer
   4. Administrator

5. A set of records that lists each monetary transaction of the facility is normally referred to as _____. (p. 183)
   1. The books
   2. Financial statements
   3. Monetary records
   4. Income and revenue statement

6. The primary purpose of the Generally Accepted Accounting Principles is to _____. (p. 183)
   1. Guarantee honesty among providers
   2. Maximize comparability of financial statements of different organizations
   3. Create a single view among financial managers
   4. Protect the owners

7. An owner who takes unrecorded cash from the facility daily cash intake to purchase a laptop for his daughter to use at college has violated the _____ concept. (pp. 183–184)
   1. Consistency
   2. Entity
   3. Time period
   4. Objective evidence

8. Instructing the financial manager to record assets at current market value and to not record patient bills expected to become uncollectible violates the _____ concept. (pp. 183–184)
   1. Entity
   2. Good faith
   3. Time period
   4. Consistency

9. Telling the accountant not to record overtime paid from the cash box to employees working weekends is violating the _____ concept. (pp. 183–184)
   1. Ongoing concern
   2. Entity
   3. Full disclosure
   4. Time period

10. Directing the accountant to move from a January 1 date to a June 30 fiscal year date in order to minimize the negative image possibly created by an anticipated loss violates the _____ concept. (pp. 183–184)
    1. Ongoing concern
    2. Time period
    3. Conservation
    4. Entity

11. Allowing the bookkeeper to destroy vouchers showing payments made for meals to employees once these are recorded may violate the _____ concept. (pp. 183–184)
    1. Objective evidence
    2. Consistency
    3. Time period
    4. Entity

12. Pieces of paper indicating money owed to or by the facility, bank statements, and similar pieces of paper or its electronic equivalent are known as _____. (p. 184)
    1. Paper trail
    2. Source documents
    3. Bill of lading
    4. Records

**13.** An administrator who instructs the accountant to begin reporting facility finances by recording all expenditures and all receipts as they actually occur has decided to use the _____ system of accounting. (pp. 184–185)
1. Cash
2. Implied
3. No-fault
4. Accrual

**14.** It is difficult to recognize items such as depreciation and prepaid insurance in the _____ system of accounting. (pp. 184–185)
1. Accrual
2. Simplified
3. Cash
4. Income and expense

**15.** An administrator directing the accountant to record revenues when they are earned and expenses when they are incurred, regardless of the time the cash transaction takes place, has decided to use the _____ approach to accounting. (pp. 184–185)
1. Accrual
2. Cash
3. Simplified
4. Advanced

**16.** Allowing the facility to accurately measure revenues earned after expenses have been paid or losses incurred by matching revenues and expenses for each time period is the advantage of the _____ system of accounting. (pp. 184–185)
1. Accrual
2. Cash
3. Income and loss
4. Advanced electronic

**17.** A summary of the nursing home's financial well-being within a time period is normally referred to as _____. (p. 187)
1. The financial statements
2. Profit and loss
3. Notes to changes in financial condition
4. Statements of change

**18.** If the administrator asked the bookkeeper for a list containing every account in the facility, the bookkeeper would hand the administrator the _____. (p. 187)
1. Books
2. Financial report
3. Chart of accounts
4. General journal

**19.** Things owned by the facility are normally referred to as (p. 187)
1. Debentures
2. Assets
3. Possessions
4. Tangibles

**20.** Things owed by the facility, its obligations, are normally referred to as ____. (p. 187)
1. Capital
2. Unpaid bills
3. Invoices
4. Liabilities

**21.** Money invested in the facility, also known as the facility's net worth, is normally referred to as ____. (p. 187)
1. Stock
2. Collateral
3. Capital
4. Income stream

**22.** If the administrator asks the accountant for the journals, the administrator wants to look at ____. (p. 188)
1. The original entries
2. The assets
3. The debits
4. Current summaries of income and outgo

**23.** The new accountant informs the administrator that to simplify things, he has incorporated all purchases that will be paid for the next few years into the accounts payable journal. The administrator should ____. (p. 188)
1. Compliment the accountant
2. Ask for last year's books to be conformed to the new system
3. Begin a search for a new accountant
4. Ask that these purchases be transferred to the general journal

**24.** Making a debit and a credit entry for each transaction is known as the ____ system of accounting. (pp. 188–191)
1. Single/double
2. Systematic
3. Alternate
4. Double-entry

**25.** Under double-entry bookkeeping, when a bill is sent to Ms. Jones for $3,000 for the past month's care, the bookkeeper would normally record $3,000 in the debit column as an increase in assets and (pp. 188–191)
1. Record $3,000 on the credit side as an increase in revenue
2. Record $3,000 as received
3. Wait for the payment before entering further data
4. Enter an estimate of when the bill will be paid

**26.** Using accrual accounting, purchase of a 6-month supply of provisions would be entered into the ____. (p. 192)
1. Billings journal
2. Cash receipts journal
3. General journal
4. Credit side of the ledger

27. Under accrual accounting, when the accountant shows the amount of medical supplies used during a month in the cash disbursements journal and the general journal the bookkeeper has made _____. (p. 192)
    1. A mistake
    2. An adjusting entry
    3. An inappropriate entry
    4. A good accounting judgment

28. When errors are discovered in other journals, they can be corrected by entries into the _____. (p. 192)
    1. Support records
    2. Ledger
    3. Cash receipts journal
    4. General journal

29. When the administrator asks the accountant for a summary of all debits and credits contained in the journals for the time period, the accountant should hand the _____ to the administrator. (p. 192)
    1. General journal
    2. General ledger
    3. Financial statements
    4. Debits and credits listing

30. At the end of a time period, when debits do not match credits exactly, the accountant can first assume an error has been made in _____. (p. 193)
    1. Recording transactions
    2. Entering debits
    3. Entering credits
    4. Source documents

31. The GAAPs do not normally require financial statements prepared for general distribution to include _____. (p. 193)
    1. Income statement, or profit/loss statement
    2. Balance sheet, or statement of financial position
    3. Statement of changes in financial position
    4. Chart of accounts

32. The income statement shows whether _____ were sufficient to cover expenses. (p. 193)
    1. Charges
    2. Revenues
    3. Debts
    4. Retained earnings

33. The accountant has listed the new building annex, the new central air conditioning system, and the supplies for the next 6 months as capital expenses. The administrator should _____. (pp. 193–194)
    1. Be pleased with the decisions
    2. Forward the report to corporate headquarters
    3. Rewrite the report
    4. Look for a new accountant

**34.** At the end of a time period, total expenses are subtracted from total revenues to compute the _____. (p. 194)
   *1.* Net income, or profit or loss
   *2.* Approximate income
   *3.* Adjusted income margin
   *4.* Operating income

**35.** The accountant, upon successfully bringing the expense and revenue accounts to zero, has successfully (p. 197)
   *1.* Calculated profit
   *2.* Calculated losses
   *3.* Closed the books
   *4.* Completed the financial statements

**36.** When the administrator asks the chief financial officer for a statement showing the ending balance of the revenue and expense accounts, the CFO should hand the _____ to the administrator. (p. 197)
   *1.* Income statement
   *2.* Balance sheet
   *3.* General ledger
   *4.* General journal

**37.** A financial statement in which the assets must equal the liability and capital accounts is known as the _____. (p. 197)
   *1.* Ending statement
   *2.* Final statement
   *3.* Balance sheet
   *4.* Financial statement

**38.** Any possession of the facility which will be or could be turned into cash within 12 months is a _____. (p. 199)
   *1.* Noncurrent asset
   *2.* Current asset
   *3.* Benefit
   *4.* Positive asset

**39.** The concept that, since capital assets will not be liquidated any time soon, their current market value is not directly relevant, relates to the ongoing concern concept and is known as _____. (p. 199)
   *1.* Historic cost
   *2.* Current cost
   *3.* Original cost
   *4.* Projected value

**40.** Depreciation is an expense associated with the use of _____. (p. 199)
   *1.* A purchase
   *2.* An asset
   *3.* Land
   *4.* A specified purchase

**41.** Bills from suppliers of foodstuffs or office supplies, or janitorial services contractors are normally classified as among the _____. (p. 199)
   *1.* Current liabilities
   *2.* Accounts due
   *3.* Invoices
   *4.* Bills of lading

**42.** When an administrator notes that there are $600,000 in notes payable on the financial reports, she knows these must be paid within _____. (p. 199)
   *1.* 6 months
   *2.* 1 year
   *3.* 1 month
   *4.* 90 days

**43.** Funds that have been put into the facility by owners or others, and retained earnings that have been put back into the facility are usually included when calculating the _____. (p. 199)
   *1.* Net worth
   *2.* Bottom line
   *3.* Final value
   *4.* Financial liabilities

**44.** If the administrator asks the accountant for a statement analyzing the financial position of the facility at the beginning of the fiscal year, the best statement to hand the administrator is the _____. (p. 199)
   *1.* Statement of profit and loss
   *2.* Statement of net worth
   *3.* Balance sheet
   *4.* General ledger

**45.** The certified public accountant's end of year report for a 15-year-old, 120-bed for-profit facility with no debt shows an excess of income over expenses of $95,000. The owners would likely be _____. (p. 200)
   *1.* Very pleased with facility performance
   *2.* Very displeased with facility performance
   *3.* Generally satisfied
   *4.* Neutral

**46.** When asked whether funds are readily available for a $75,000, purchase and the accountant responds that the net worth is well over $800,000 and to go ahead with the purchase, the administrator should (p. 201)
   *1.* Ask for a statement of working capital
   *2.* Make the purchase
   *3.* Seek a vertical analysis
   *4.* Amortize the purchase

47. When the amount of current assets remaining after current liabilities have been subtracted is calculated, the administrator has an idea of the _____ available to be spent. (p. 201)
    1. Capital
    2. Net worth
    3. Working capital
    4. Assets

48. When the chief financial officer identifies trends in measures of the facility's financial performance by comparing the same relationships for several time periods he is doing (p. 202)
    1. Comparison analysis
    2. Time period analyses
    3. Ratio analyses
    4. Trade-off comparisons

49. A facility has current assets of $403,898 and current liabilities of $367,000. Its current ratio is _____. (p. 202)
    1. 9
    2. 3
    3. 1.1
    4. 2.1

50. A 1-year-old, 120-bed for-profit facility with a $2,500,000 mortgage at 7.4% reports a net operating margin before depreciation of $25,000. In today's financial market, the owners would likely be _____. (p. 204)
    1. Very pleased
    2. Very displeased
    3. Seeking to sell the facility as a result
    4. Seeking to refinance as a result

51. Ratios, to be truly useful, should be _____. (p. 202)
    1. Used to measure over time
    2. Compared with industry averages over time
    3. In simple mathematical terms
    4. Compared to expected future ratios

52. The new administrator in a private pay for-profit facility is told by the accountant that the accounts receivable are $105,800 and the net operating revenues are $334,000. Upon calculating the average collection period ratio, which turns out to be _____ days, the administrator should be _____. (p. 203)
    1. 29      pleased
    2. 29      displeased
    3. 115     pleased
    4. 115     upset

**53.** A 12-year-old facility, largely out of debt, has $334,693 in operating revenues and $339,078 in operating expenses, yielding a net operating margin ratio of _____. The owners of this facility would likely feel this to be _____. (p. 204)
  *1.* .013     unacceptable
  *2.* .013     acceptable
  *3.* 8.013    unacceptable
  *4.* 8.013    acceptable

**54.** A facility with long-term debt of $4,000,000 and a total equity of $3,000,000 has a debt to equity ratio of _____ , which is _____ the industry average. (p. 204)
  *1.* 1.33     considerably above
  *2.* 1.33     considerably below
  *3.* 2.33     far above
  *4.* 2.33     well below

**55.** Trends and patterns in the operation of a nursing facility can best be obtained by doing _____. (p. 205)
  *1.* Ratio analyses
  *2.* Vertical analyses
  *3.* Ratio and vertical analyses over time
  *4.* Ratio and vertical analyses

**56.** To safeguard the finances of a facility, procedures should be arranged to establish a system of _____ so that employees review each other's financial activities. (p. 207)
  *1.* Checks
  *2.* Dual bookkeeping
  *3.* Checks and balances
  *4.* Antitheft devices

**57.** A useful form that summarizes the facility's occupancy, listing daily admissions, discharges, and transfers is known as the _____. (p. 208)
  *1.* Daily census form
  *2.* Headcount
  *3.* Weekly census report
  *4.* Occupancy ratio

**58.** At the end of each year for facilities participating in Medicare, a Medicare Cost Reconciliation settlement occurs in which _____. (p. 214)
  *1.* The facility receives additional money
  *2.* The facility pays out additional money
  *3.* The facility receives or pays back money
  *4.* A flat rate per patient per month is paid the facility

**59.** The frozen food contractor arrives, places the order in the freezer, checks off the receiving slip, hands it to the appropriate kitchen employee who thanks the contractor, and hands the receiving slip and purchase order copy to the director of food services. The administrator, on observing this, should _____. (p. 215)
1. Be pleased with the smoothness of the working relationship
2. Compliment the contractor for an efficient delivery
3. Be upset
4. Continue to enjoy his/her cup of coffee

**60.** Perhaps the only way to maintain an accurate count of supplies consumed and those remaining is to use _____. (p. 218)
1. A computer program
2. A hand-counted inventory system
3. A receipt inventory system
4. A perpetual inventory system

**61.** The use of LIFO (last in first out) to price inventory during a period of inflation will have the effect of making the value of the goods remaining in inventory _____. (p. 220)
1. Higher
2. Lower
3. About the same
4. At market value

**62.** The largest directly controllable cost for the average administrator is _____. (p. 220)
1. Inventory/supplies
2. Labor
3. Long-term debt financing costs
4. Short-term debt financing costs

**63.** Payroll deductions are subtracted from _____ to arrive at the employee's _____ pay. (p. 220)
1. Net/gross
2. Total/net
3. Gross/net
4. Overall/take-home

**64.** Assets that can be capitalized or depreciated differ from the other assets of a facility in that they are used in operations for more than _____ and will not be converted into _____ within the year. (p. 224)
1. One time period/cash
2. Two time periods/debt
3. A balance sheet period/securities
4. 3 years/cash

**65.** Upon discovering that the new accountant had set the actual purchase price paid (e.g., no tax, delivery, or similar costs) for the assets to be depreciated, the facility administrator would normally feel the accountant was _____. (p. 224)
1. Sharp and on the ball
2. Not serving the facility well
3. Overestimating historical costs
4. Doing okay, all things considered

**66.** One practical reason for using straight line depreciation is that _____. (p. 225)
1. It brings the fastest write-off
2. It is the only fully acceptable method
3. Most third-party payers require it
4. It has the approval of the IRS

**67.** Congress' purpose for passing accelerated depreciation was to _____ of new facilities. (p. 225)
1. Discourage overbuilding
2. Encourage more building
3. Regulate construction
4. Deregulate construction

**68.** As a practical matter, most owners do not fund depreciation and treat it as _____. (p. 226)
1. Money available to the facility to spend
2. Money to be placed in reserve
3. A fiction
4. A useless set of required calculations

**69.** Using several differing depreciation schedules for a single piece of equipment is _____ as an accounting behavior. (p. 226)
1. Unacceptable
2. Quite acceptable
3. Risky
4. Illegal

**70.** Land _____ is a depreciable asset. (p. 226)
1. Never
2. Sometimes
3. For for-profit facilities
4. For nonprofit facilities

**71.** Medical supplies, food supplies, and postage for billing residents are _____ costs. (p. 228)
1. Fixed
2. Variable
3. Semi-variable
4. Break-even

**72.** The salary of the director of nurses and the administrator are examples of _____ costs. (p. 228)
1. Fixed
2. Variable
3. Semi-variable
4. Proportionate

**73.** In a facility having high fixed costs, the pressure to keep beds filled is _____ in facilities with low fixed costs. (p. 228)
1. About the same as
2. Stronger than
3. Weaker than
4. More moderate than

**74.** For in-facility services such as physical therapy, it is important to calculate the _____ cost in order to better analyze the cost effectiveness of such services. (pp. 229–230)
  1. Total
  2. Break-even
  3. Minimum
  4. Maximum

**75.** Nursing and physical therapy are normally thought of as _____ centers. (pp. 229–230)
  1. Cost
  2. Loss
  3. Revenue
  4. Break-even

**76.** A financial analysis that yields to the administrator a representative picture of the entire expense of providing a service (e.g., offering adult day care services) is known as _____. (p. 231)
  1. Value analysis
  2. Revenue analysis
  3. Cost ending
  4. Center analysis

**77.** Only when appropriate _____ has been achieved can an accurate job of _____ be accomplished. (p. 232)
  1. Information gathering/cost setting
  2. Cost finding/rate setting
  3. Expense reporting/estimating income
  4. Tax analysis/cost setting

**78.** In order to develop a reasonable estimate of income and expenses for a coming time period, it is important to do both a/an _____ budget and a _____ budget. (pp. 237–238)
  1. Capital cash
  2. Expense revenue
  3. Expense balanced
  4. Cash capital

**79.** Because income and expenses vary from time period to time period, it is desirable to project a _____ budget. (p. 239)
  1. Cash
  2. Balanced
  3. Forecasted
  4. Capital

**80.** Plans for expenditures for buildings, major equipment, and the like are normally part of the _____ budget. (pp. 239–240)
  1. Cash
  2. Revenue
  3. Expense
  4. Capital

81. A method of measuring the potential profitability of an investment, calculated by dividing the net income by the investment is the _____. (p. 254)
    1. Activity-based costing
    2. ARR (accounting rate of return)
    3. Profit ratio
    4. Profit assurance calculation

82. A revision of an accounting forecast or assumption about the facility's expected or experienced performance is a/an _____. (p. 254)
    1. Change in accounting estimate
    2. Change in performance
    3. Review
    4. Accountant's revision

83. The portion of a brand in the form of a symbol, design, or distinctive coloring or lettering, also called a logo, is an organization's _____. (p. 255)
    1. Intangible asset
    2. Sign
    3. Brand mark
    4. Original art

84. The administrator decides to offer newer forms of physical therapy that reduce use of currently used physical therapy methods. She has _____ the current methods. (p. 256)
    1. Reduced the competitive advantage of
    2. Cannibalized
    3. Reduced
    4. Usurped

85. A market that is so competitive that all its participants have virtually no control over price is known as _____. (p. 257)
    1. Niche marketing
    2. No holds barred competition
    3. Perfect competition
    4. Imperfect markets

86. The administrator asks the business manager to divide the net income after any taxes by the noncurrent liabilities + owners' equity. He wants the _____. (p. 258)
    1. Best income estimate
    2. Return on invested capital estimate
    3. Probability estimate
    4. Best productivity achievable

87. A method of determining the optimum amount of materials that needs to be ordered on a regular basis is known as the _____. (p. 258)
    1. Best ordering method
    2. Ordering queue
    3. Economic order quantity
    4. Inventory control procedure

88. When governments use their powers to keep the price either above or below the equilibrium point it is known as _____. (p. 260)
   1. Market interference
   2. Government control
   3. Price controls
   4. Government rule

89. Short-term securities (2 days to 270 days) issued by corporations, banks, and other borrowing institutions to raise short-term working capital is known as _____. (p. 261)
   1. Securities fraud
   2. Commercial paper
   3. Short-term bonds
   4. Notes payable

90. The administrator asks the bank for an instrument stating that that bank that has granted the holder the amount of credit equal to the face amount wants a _____. (p. 261)
   1. Short-term loan
   2. Long-term loan
   3. Letter of credit
   4. Letter of assurance

91. The facility has issued a debt obligation to pay a specific amount on a stated date. The facility has issued _____. (p. 261)
   1. Letters of credit
   2. Notes
   3. Bonds
   4. Financial instruments

92. When the financial manager classifies an expense as an asset because it benefits the facility for more than 1 year he has _____ that expense. (p. 261)
   1. Adjusted
   2. Reduced
   3. Spread
   4. Capitalized

93. The administrator wishes to lease a building and acquire substantial property rights in the process. She seeks _____. (p. 262)
   1. A leasehold
   2. A long-term lease
   3. A capital lease
   4. Refinancing

94. The administrator has borrowed cash for an agreed upon purpose between a lender and borrower. He now has a _____. (p. 262)
   1. Legal obligation
   2. Bond
   3. Note
   4. Capital asset

95. The chain issues stocks and bonds that can be converted into capital stock at some future date. They have issued _____. (p. 263)
    1. Convertible bonds
    2. Convertible securities
    3. Quasi-bonds
    4. Quasi-bonds and quasi-stocks

96. The chain "buys back" a portion of its outstanding stock by giving one new share in place of each four previously held shares. The chain has accomplished a/an _____. (p. 263)
    1. Reverse split
    2. Buy-back
    3. Buy-down
    4. Illegal move

97. The administrator seeks to be licensed without having to meet all the conditions new entrants would have to meet. She seeks to be _____. (p. 264)
    1. Grandfathered
    2. Granted concessions
    3. Avoiding current requirements
    4. Advancing herself

98. The administrator holds a number of assets, such as bonds or easily sold stock, as investments. He has substantial _____. (p. 264)
    1. Sources of income
    2. Riches
    3. Good investments
    4. Cash equivalents

99. The instrument that creates a corporation under the laws of a state is known as the _____. (p. 265)
    1. Registration
    2. Certificate
    3. Statement of incorporation
    4. Articles of incorporation

100. The three owners hold all the shares in the facility. They have a _____. (p. 265)
    1. Cash cow
    2. Profitable operation
    3. Semipublic corporation
    4. Privately held company

## LEGAL AND BUSINESS TERMINOLOGY: SOURCES OF LAW, THE COURT SYSTEMS

1. Statutes are laws _____. (p. 241)
    1. Known as common law
    2. Made by judges
    3. Passed by cities
    4. Passed by legislatures

2. Normally, courts of appeal do not have _____. (p. 242)
   1. Criminal jurisdiction
   2. Original jurisdiction
   3. Criminal law enforcement authority
   4. Authority to hear misdemeanors

3. Statutes and subsequent regulations are collected in _____. (p. 241)
   1. The Code
   2. Constitutional amendments
   3. The Federal Requirements
   4. Law books

4. Generally, the lowest level of the court system is the _____ court. (p. 242)
   1. Circuit
   2. Criminal
   3. Civil
   4. Magistrate's

## LEGAL TERMINOLOGY

5. To set a person or corporation free of accusations is to _____. (p. 242)
   1. Enjoin
   2. Acquit
   3. Consent
   4. Motion

6. A statement in writing given under oath before a notary public is an _____. (p. 243)
   1. Affidavit
   2. Affirmation
   3. Appeal
   4. Appearance

7. The coming into court of a person being summoned to do so is a/an _____. (p. 243)
   1. Appeal
   2. Discovery
   3. Appearance
   4. Injunction

8. An impartial person chosen by the parties to an argument who agree to abide by her decision is a/an _____. (p. 243)
   1. Arbitrator
   2. Adjudicator
   3. Civil judge
   4. Attorney at law

9. A Latin phrase meaning to stand by earlier court decisions is _____. (p. 245)
   1. Stare decisis
   2. Res judicata
   3. Res ipsa loquitur
   4. Respondeat superior

**10.** A verdict, given by a jury at the direction of a judge is a/an (p. 244)
1. Directed verdict
2. Dismissal
3. Indictment
4. Injunction

**11.** An application to the court asking for an action favorable to one's side is _____. (p. 245)
1. A witnessing
2. A motion
3. An application to the court
4. A plea bargain

**12.** When the employee is acting within the control or scope of the employer, the employer is responsible for the acts of the employee under the concept of _____. (p. 246)
1. Contractor-employee relations
2. Strict liability
3. A subcontractor relationship
4. Borrowed servant

**13.** A written publication that exposes someone to public scorn, hatred, con-tempt, or ridicule is _____. (p. 246)
1. Libel
2. Slander
3. An aggrieved party
4. An assault

**14.** An early step in a criminal procedure during which the defendant is formally charged with an offense is a/an _____. (p. 246)
1. Discovery
2. Arraignment
3. Adjudication
4. Action

**15.** Conduct giving rise to a cause for legal action is _____. (p. 246)
1. Actionable
2. An adjudication
3. An appeal
4. An indictment

**16.** When parties to a lawsuit who are dissatisfied with the court's decision ask a higher court to review the decision, it is known as a/an _____. (p. 246)
1. Appeal
2. Arbitration
3. Respondeat superior
4. Stare decisis

**17.** A district attorney may bring assault charges for the purpose of _____. (p. 246)
1. Revenge
2. Punishment
3. Monetary award
4. Defamation

**18.** Damages for proven losses are known as _____ damages. (p. 244)
   *1.* Actual
   *2.* Exemplary
   *3.* Incidental
   *4.* Punitive

**19.** A fee paid in advance to an attorney for services on a case is known as a _____. (p. 245)
   *1.* Lien
   *2.* Prepayment
   *3.* Retainer
   *4.* Reward

**20.** A concept in torts used as a defense by the defendant against the plaintiff is an assumption of _____ (p. 244)
   *1.* Risk
   *2.* Innocence
   *3.* Guilt
   *4.* Fraud

**21.** Consent given after full information regarding the matter has been provided is known as _____ consent. (p. 243)
   *1.* Informed
   *2.* Individual
   *3.* Intended
   *4.* Personal

**22.** Spoken statements leading to actual damages implying crime, unchastity, or relating to a person's profession or business is known as _____. (p. 244)
   *1.* Libel
   *2.* Slander
   *3.* Exemplary damages
   *4.* Consequential damages

**23.** A reckless disregard for human life, a state of mind that accompanies a wrongful act in which the resulting harm was intended, is known as _____. (p. 245)
   *1.* Malice
   *2.* Comparative negligence
   *3.* A heinous act
   *4.* Contempt

**24.** A public official, either elected or appointed, who conducts cases against persons accused of crimes is known as a _____. (p. 245)
   *1.* Lawyer
   *2.* Prosecutor
   *3.* Judge
   *4.* Bailiff

**25.** A written order from a judge permitting certain law enforcement officers to look for certain things or persons is a _____. (p. 246)
1. Retainer
2. Search certificate
3. Search and rescue
4. Search warrant

**26.** A person who gives evidence before a court and swears that testimony is true is a _____. (p. 246)
1. Clerk of court
2. Bailiff
3. Sheriff
4. Witness

**27.** A _____ exists when a legal duty is owed another, that duty is breached, and harm results. (p. 246)
1. Tort
2. Lien
3. Deposition
4. Warrant

**28.** A written order from a judge having authority in that jurisdiction for the arrest of a person is known as a _____. (p. 247)
1. Tort
2. Summons
3. Warrant
4. Directed verdict

## RISKS ASSUMED BY THE OPERATION OF A LONG-TERM CARE FACILITY

**29.** Concept, in both civil and criminal law, that the employer is responsible without the employee having to show employer fault, and normally applying to an ultra hazardous situations is _____. (p. 247)
1. Scope of employment
2. Respondeat superior
3. Contractor
4. Strict liability

**30.** The range of employee activities held by the courts to be the legal responsibility of the employer, essentially any act performed in the process of carrying out one's duties, is known as _____. (p. 248)
1. Scope of employment
2. Range of job activities
3. Employee job assignments
4. Zone of employment

**31.** Laws that generally establish employer responsibility without regard to fault or negligence for employees' illness or injuries that arise out of performance of the job are known as _____. (p. 248)
1. Worker's Compensation Act
2. Employer's Liability Act
3. Worker Insurance Program
4. Worker Protection Act

**32.** Statutes in various states setting forth the extent to which employers are liable in regard to their employees are _____. (p. 247)
1. Employer's Liability Acts
2. Borrowed Servant Acts
3. Contractor Acts
4. Employee's Rights Laws

# 4

# NAB Domain: Environment

# Learning the Continuum of Long-Term Care

## INDUSTRY OVERVIEW

1.  During the years 1993–2008, the percentage of chain-owned nursing facilities _____. (p. 284)
    1.  Was about 5%
    2.  Varied between just under and just over half
    3.  Doubled
    4.  Tripled

2.  During the years 1993–2008, the occupancy rates for U.S. nursing facilities _____. (p. 284)
    1.  Remained unchanged
    2.  Decreased
    3.  Continued to increase slightly
    4.  Increased as hospital discharge rates spiked

3.  As a result of few new nursing homes being built in recent decades it can be expected that occupancy rates in nursing home _____ over the next 30 years. (pp. 283–284)
    1.  Will remain level
    2.  Will decrease
    3.  May decrease
    4.  Will be near 100%

4.  The projections of daily volume of long-term care assistance by all categories of caregivers is expected to _____. (p. 280)
    1.  Increase marginally
    2.  Steadily increase
    3.  Decrease as older persons get healthier
    4.  Decrease

**5.** The projections of daily volume of long-term care assistance needed in the year 2040 is about _____ the need identified in 1980. (p. 280)
1. Equal to
2. Twice
3. Three times
4. Four times

**6.** Percentage of Medicaid dollars spent on institutional care, over the past couple of decades, has _____ (p. 293)
1. Increased dramatically
2. Decreased slightly
3. Been unchanged
4. Doubled

**7.** The American Association of Homes and Services for the Aging is the _____. (p. 298)
1. National for-profit group
2. National nonprofit group
3. Federal regional authority
4. National federal authority

**8.** The proportion of Medicare nursing home residents who, at any one time reside in facilities, is _____ the proportion who are Medicaid. (p. 307)
1. About equal to
2. Far smaller than
3. Far larger than
4. Larger and growing

## MEDICARE AND MEDICAID

**1.** The federal government matches state expenditures ranging from _____. (p. 300)
1. 50% to 83%
2. 50% to 95%
3. 40% to 60%
4. 25% to 45%

**2.** In 2008 the federal government changed the "look back" period for which Medicaid assistance may be denied due to "gifts" _____. (p. 307)
1. To cover only the medically indigent
2. To relax the rules
3. To provide relief to middle class elderly
4. From 3 years to 5 years look back

## THE LIFE SAFETY CODE

**3.** The *Life Safety Code* _____. (p. 338)
1. Is too often ignored by states
2. Must be used in every state
3. Is fully voluntary for cities and counties
4. Has the effect of law in most states

4. An employee hearing the fire code phrase must _____. (p. 340)
   1. Exit the facility
   2. Help fellow employees as needed
   3. Go to his station
   4. Ask nearby persons where the fire is located

5. Under the *Life Safety Code®,* movement of infirm patients to safe areas or the exterior is _____ in fire drills. (p. 340)
   1. Required
   2. Not required
   3. At the option of the local fire chief
   4. Optional

6. On discovery of fire involving a person, personnel shall immediately _____. (p. 340)
   1. Assist the person
   2. Transmit a fire alarm
   3. Aid the person and call aloud "fire"
   4. Aid the person while calling aloud an established code phrase

7. Basic action required of health care facility personnel are _____. (p. 340)
   1. Removal of directly involved occupants
   2. Transmission of an alarm signal
   3. Confinement of the effects of the fire
   4. All of the above

8. Often the most dangerous element threatening patient safety is _____. (p. 340)
   1. Unavailability of correct type of extinguisher
   2. Slow thinking responses by personnel
   3. Smoke inhalation
   4. First- and second-degree burns

9. Smoking by residents classified as "not responsible" shall be prohibited except _____. (pp. 340–341)
   1. Under exceptional circumstances (e.g., terminal illness)
   2. Under medical direction
   3. When the resident is under direct supervision
   4. When other residents agree to permit smoking

10. The overall objective of the *Life Safety Code* for new health care occupancies is to (p. 339)
    1. Limit spread of a fire to the room of fire origin
    2. Require sprinkler systems or their equivalent as applicable
    3. Educate the public on correct fire procedures
    4. Provide guidelines for the local fire chief

11. Facility personnel that shall be instructed in the use of and response to fire alarm include _____. (p. 340)
    1. Nursing staff
    2. All staff having patient contact
    3. Nursing and dietary staff
    4. All personnel

**12.** When a facility locks exits it must _____. (p. 340)
   *1.* Hire additional staff
   *2.* Use special locks
   *3.* Get permission from the local fire marshal
   *4.* Maintain adequate staff to release locks

**13.** A material that, in the form in which it is used, will not aid combustion or add appreciable heat to spreading fire is defined as _____. (p. 341)
   *1.* Fire-resistant
   *2.* Fire-coded
   *3.* Noncombustible
   *4.* Combustible

**14.** In determining occupant loads in exit requirements, the actual expected count or a projection using _____ square feet of floor space in sleeping areas and _____ square feet of floor space in treatment areas shall be used. (p. 343)
   *1.* 120      240
   *2.* 100      200
   *3.* 220      440
   *4.* 440      640

**15.** Handrails clearance from the wall must be at least _____. (p. 345)
   *1.* 1 hand wide
   *2.* 6 inches
   *3.* 1 and one-half inches
   *4.* 8 inches

**16.** The purpose of smokeproof towers is to _____. (p. 345)
   *1.* Limit infiltration of heat, smoke, and fire gases
   *2.* Contain construction costs
   *3.* Improve the visual appeal of the building
   *4.* Totally eliminate smoke and gases

**17.** The National Safety Council has suggested slopes of 7 to 20 degrees for a _____. (p. 345)
   *1.* Stairway
   *2.* Stairway and landings
   *3.* Stairway and ramp
   *4.* Ramp

**18.** Aisles, corridors, and ramps used for exit must be at least _____ in width, clear, and unobstructed. (p. 345)
   *1.* 8 feet
   *2.* 3 feet
   *3.* Within residents' ability to move
   *4.* Reasonably wide

**19.** Travel distance within a room to an exit must not exceed _____. (pp. 345–346)
   *1.* 25 yards
   *2.* 50 feet
   *3.* Good judgment
   *4.* Local fire marshal rules

**20.** Each floor or fire section of the facility shall have at least _____ located _____ from each other. (p. 346)
1. Three exits/remotely
2. Two exits/remotely
3. Two ramps/away
4. Three ramps/remotely

**21.** Travel distance from within any patient room to an exit access must not exceed _____. (p. 346)
1. 50 feet
2. 75 feet
3. 100 feet
4. 200 feet

**22.** Illumination of the means of egress must be continuous and must provide at least _____ foot-candle(s) measured at the _____. (p. 346)
1. 1 floor
2. 2 railings
3. 1 railing
4. 2 floor

**23.** The emergency lighting system must provide power _____. (p. 346)
1. Automatically
2. With a minimum of operations
3. From each nursing station
4. From a switch in the administrator's office

**24.** Exit signs must be placed so that a person is never more than _____ from the nearest exit sign. (p. 346)
1. 50 feet
2. 100 feet
3. 150 feet
4. 200 feet

**25.** Corridors throughout patient sleeping areas must have _____. (p. 347)
1. Automatic smoke detection systems
2. 9 feet in clearance
3. Well decorated walls
4. Smooth surfaces

**26.** A supervised automatic sprinkler system _____. (p. 347)
1. Is advised
2. Should be installed
3. Is a luxury for the average nursing facility
4. Is required

**27.** Short persons must be able to reach _____ (p. 348)
1. Fire extinguishers
2. Door stops
3. Top shelves
4. Top of bureaus

**28.** A fixed, regularly serviced, automatic fire extinguishing system in nursing home kitchens over the cook stoves is _____. (p. 347)
1. Required
2. Permitted in most states
3. Highly recommended
4. Optional

**29.** Every building shall have a/an _____ operated fire alarm system that shall be _____ supervised. (p. 347)
1. Sprinkler continuously
2. Automatic continuously
3. Simultaneously continuously
4. Manually electronically

**30.** Every story used by patients must be divided into (p. 348)
1. Four smoke compartments
2. Equal spaces
3. Two smoke compartments
4. Five smoke compartments

**31.** Every story with 50 or more occupants must be divided into at least _____. (p. 348)
1. Six rooms
2. Two smoke compartments
3. Two nursing stations responsibilities
4. Four smoke compartments

**32.** Extinguishers should be checked _____ by the fire department and recharged and serviced _____ by a qualified person. (pp. 347–348)
1. Monthly monthly
2. Monthly quarterly
3. Monthly annually
4. Quarterly annually

**33.** Doors protecting corridor openings must be made of 1¾ inches solid bonded core wood or constructed to resist fire for at least _____ minutes. (p. 348)
1. 10
2. 20
3. 60
4. 45

**34.** Each patient room must have an outside window or door. If a window, it _____. (p. 348)
1. Must be at least 2 feet by 4 feet
2. Must have a latch on it
3. Need not be operable
4. Must be thermopane

## AMERICANS WITH DISABILITIES ACT

**35.** For changes in level: up to ¼ inch is _____ , between ¼ and ½ inch _____ is required, and over ½ inch must meet _____ requirements. (p. 352)
   *1.* Permissible/beveled edge/ramp
   *2.* Ignored/curved edge/grade
   *3.* Permitted/sharp edge/ramp
   *4.* Required/rounded edge/grade

**36.** On any given flight of stairs, riser heights and tread widths must be _____. (p. 352)
   *1.* Uniform
   *2.* Appropriate
   *3.* Approved
   *4.* Cleared with the architect

**37.** High forward reach limit is generally _____. (p. 352)
   *1.* 5 feet
   *2.* 6 feet
   *3.* 48 inches
   *4.* Up to the facility to determine

**38.** Minimum width for two wheelchairs to pass is _____ inches. (p. .353)
   *1.* 40
   *2.* 60
   *3.* 72
   *4.* 82

**39.** Side reach should be between _____ inches off the floor. (p. 352)
   *1.* 9 and 54
   *2.* 20 and 40
   *3.* 60 and 70
   *4.* 12 and 24

**40.** Handrails must extend at least _____ inches beyond a ramp or stair and be parallel to the floor or ground surface. (p. 354)
   *1.* 4
   *2.* 6
   *3.* 8
   *4.* 12

**41.** The generally specified maximum pounds of pressure required to operate doors, windows, and so on, is _____. (p. 365)
   *1.* 1
   *2.* 3
   *3.* 5
   *4.* 10

**42.** Automatic doors and power-assisted doors should be slow-opening and low-pow-ered, not opening back to back faster than _____ seconds nor with a force of more than _____ pounds. (p. 360)
1. 3/15
2. 5/20
3. 10/30
4. 15/45

**43.** Grab bars located between _____ and _____ inches high must be provided for toi-lets on the side and back walls. (p. 368)
1. 33/36
2. 30/40
3. 20/40
4. 25/45

**44.** Grab bars and handrails are to be _____ to _____ inches in diameter or width, with _____ inches space between handrail and wall, and a sheer stress point of _____ pounds or greater. (p. 368)
1. 1, 2, 2, 200
2. 1¼, 1½, 1½, 250
3. ?, 4, 6, 500
4. 4, 4, 6, 600

**45.** The maximum allowable emergency alarm level is _____ decibels. (p. 368)
1. 60
2. 80
3. 100
4. 120

**46.** The general requirement for knee clearance under tables, work surfaces, sinks, and lavatories is _____. (p. 367)
1. 10 inches
2. 19 inches
3. 1 foot
4. 2 feet

## MANAGEMENT AND LABOR LEGISLATION AND REGULATIONS

**47.** Title 7 of the civil rights act of 1964 prohibited employers from discriminating on the basis of _____ (p. 312)
1. All of the below
2. Race
3. Color
4. Sex

**48.** In 1935, a major labor group emerged called the _____. (p. 316)
1. CIO (Congress of Industrial Organizations)
2. AFL (American Federation of Labor)
3. AFL-CIO
4. National Unions Group

**49.** By 1947, unions represented about 31% of the workforce. In 1990, union membership represented about ____% of the total work force. (p. 317)
1. 8
2. 16
3. 30
4. 40

**50.** The Taft-Hartley Act prohibited managers from _____. (p. 317)
1. Giving tenure to employees to discourage unionization
2. Giving wage increases to discourage unionization
3. Firing employees who give testimony under the Wagner Act
4. All of the above

**51.** The National Labor Relations Board does not _____. (p. 317)
1. Determine what the bargaining units shall be
2. Conduct representative elections by secret ballot
3. Investigate unfair labor practices
4. Make court decisions

**52.** In 1973, the hospitals and nursing facility interests did not seek _____. (p. 319)
1. Exemption from NLRB oversight
2. Priority for NLRB actions on disputes
3. Mandatory mediation requirements
4. Limit on number of bargaining units

**53.** In 1984, the NLRB favored nursing home managers by ruling that the appropriate bargaining unit is _____. (p. 320)
1. All professionals, all nonprofessional
2. Some professionals, all nonprofessional
3. Most professionals, most nonprofessional
4. Workers, managers

**54.** Discrimination was interpreted initially by the courts as harmful action, later, unequal treatment, and more recently as _____. (p. 322)
1. Unequal or adverse impact
2. Unjustifiable
3. Rule of the 1980s
4. Wrongdoing

**55.** The Civil Rights Act is enforced _____. (p. 322)
1. By the Equal Opportunities Commission
2. By the Equal Employment Commission
3. By the Equal Employment Opportunity Commission
4. Solely by the federal courts

**56.** The Fair Labor Standards Act requires that an overtime rate of _____ times the hourly (or other basis) be paid for all hours over _____ during the week. (p. 329)
1. 2/40
2. 1½/40
3. 2/35
4. 2/45

**57.** Minors under 16 may not be employed in the nursing facility except under _____.
(p. 331)
1. Temporary conditions
2. Parental consent (must be written)
3. Situations of clear need
4. A temporary permit issued by the Department of Labor

**58.** Funds for unemployment compensation come from a _____ payroll tax based on wages of each employee up to a certain _____. (p. 332)
1. State minimum
2. Federal minimum
3. Federal maximum
4. Local maximum

**59.** Under ERISA (Employee Retirement Income Security Act of 1975) employers _____ pension plan. (p. 333)
1. Are required to offer a
2. Are not required to offer a
3. Must enlarge their existing
4. Are prohibited from offering a

## THE OCCUPATIONAL SAFETY AND HEALTH ACT (OSHA)

**60.** Knowing the OSHA standards applicable to a facility is the responsibility of the (p. 335)
1. OSHA board
2. Employer (the administrator)
3. State Enforcement Commission
4. Staff

**61.** OSHA inspectors examine the records of illnesses and injuries to the _____. (p. 335)
1. Residents
2. Employees
3. Supervisors
4. Residents and the employees

**62.** Accidents and illnesses requiring first aid and not resulting in work loss _____ reported. (p. 336)
1. Do not have to be
2. Must be
3. Should be
4. Must always be

## HEALTH PLANNING

**63.** In states where a local health planning agency believes a shortage of nursing home beds exists, it may _____. (p. 377)
1. Require additional beds be built
2. Let a contract for building new beds
3. Advertise for bids
4. Issue a certificate of need

## JOINT COMMISSION ON ACCREDITATION OF HEALTHCARE ORGANIZATIONS (JCAHO)

**64.** For nursing facilities, meeting requirements set by the JCAHO is _____. (p. 378)
1. Voluntary
2. Mandatory
3. Required for Medicaid payments
4. Required for Medicare payments

# 5

# NAB Domain: Patient/
# Resident Care

# Building Your Resident
# Care Skills

## THE AGING PROCESS: OVERVIEW AND THEORIES

1. Which of the following is a safe generalization about aging? (p. 384)
   1. Old age ain't for sissies
   2. Aging is highly individualized
   3. Senility is inevitable
   4. Aging leads to dependency status

2. Professionals who study aging and are normally not physicians are called _____.
   (p. 384)
   1. Geriatricians
   2. Gerontologists
   3. Family practitioners
   4. Specialists

3. The progressive loss of cortical neurons (brain cells) and brain weight means that older persons _____ (p. 384)
   1. Begin to move more slowly
   2. Think less clearly
   3. Behave less predictably
   4. Are unaffected by the loss

4. Aging is a gradual decline of at least some of the systems in the body, which proceed _____. (p. 384)
   1. At different rates in different individuals
   2. At essentially the same rate for everyone
   3. At a rate unique to men and a rate unique to women
   4. Rapidly

5. According to Leonard Hayflick's theory, aging occurs because of _____ (p. 384)
   1. A limit of about 50 divisions for certain key groups of cells in humans
   2. Loss of collagen
   3. Wear and tear
   4. Progressive failure of the immune system

6.  According to the autoimmune response theory of aging, "copying errors" in repeated cell divisions result in cells that are progressively not recognized by the body, leading to _____. (p. 387)
    1. Triggering the immune system to attack these cells
    2. Damage to the RNA
    3. Limited cell divisions
    4. Reduction in elasticity of vital body parts, such as the blood vessels

## MEDICAL AND RELATED TERMS

## Specializations

1.  Physicians who specialize in treating older persons are _____. (p. 390)
    1. Gerontologists
    2. Family doctors
    3. Geriatricians
    4. Specialists

2.  A physician who diagnoses and treats diseases of the brain, nervous system, and spinal cord is a/an _____. (p. 390)
    1. Ophthalmologist
    2. Optician
    3. Optometrist
    4. Neurologist

3.  A technician, not a physician, trained to grind and to fit lenses is a/an_____. (p. 390)
    1. General surgeon
    2. Orthopedist
    3. Ophthalmologist
    4. Optician

4.  A dentist who specializes in the extraction of teeth is a/an _____. (p. 390)
    1. Osteopath
    2. Orthopedist
    3. Exodontists
    4. Periodontist

5.  A physician who specializes in diagnostic procedures and treatment of nonsurgical cases is known as a/an _____. (p. 390)
    1. Orthopedist
    2. Urologist
    3. Internist
    4. Externist

6.  A physician who specializes in examination of body tissues under laboratory conditions is known as a/an _____. (p. 390)
    1. Podiatrist
    2. Pathologist
    3. Internist
    4. Specialist

7. A physician who specializes in physical medicine, body movements, and conditioning is known as a _____. (p. 390)
   1. Pedodontist
   2. Pediatrician
   3. Physiatrist
   4. Podiatrist

8. A physician who specializes in the diagnosis and treatment of mental disorders is
   known as a/an _____. (p. 391)
   1. Psychiatrist
   2. Psychologist
   3. Psychic advisor
   4. Exodontist

9. A physician specializing in the use of X-ray and similar medical diagnostic machines
   is known as a/an _____. (p. 391)
   1. Radiologist
   2. Anesthesiologist
   3. Cardiologist
   4. Chiropractor

10. A psychiatrist who specializes in the use of psychoanalytic techniques of therapy is
    known as a/an _____. (p. 391)
    1. Psychoanalyst
    2. Psychologist
    3. Pathologist
    4. Endocrinologist

11. A physician specializing in the diagnosis and treatment of the large intestine, par-
    ticularly the rectum, is known as a/an _____ (p. 391)
    1. Optometrist
    2. Podiatrist
    3. Proctologist
    4. Allergist

12. A physician specializing in treatment of the kidney and bladder is known as a/an
    _____. (p. 391)
    1. Exodontist
    2. Urologist
    3. Periodontist
    4. Proctologist

13. A physician who specializes in the treatment of arthritic diseases is known as
    a/an _____ (p. 391)
    1. Pedodontist
    2. Rheumatologist
    3. Orthodontist
    4. Orthopedist

14. A physician specializing in the treatment of the lungs is known as a/an _____. (p. 391)
    1. Pulmonologist
    2. Periodontist
    3. Plastic surgeon
    4. Dental specialist

15. A physician who diagnoses and treats eye diseases and disorders, performs eye surgery, refracts the eyes, and prescribes corrective eyeglasses and lenses is known as a/an _____. (p. 390)
    1. Optician
    2. Ophthalmologist
    3. Neurosurgeon
    4. Osteopath

## Therapeutic Actions of Drugs

1. Induces vomiting, for example, warm salt water: _____. (pp. 396–397)
    1. Antiemetic
    2. Emetic
    3. Sedative
    4. Hypotensive drug

2. Destroys tissue by local application, for example, silver nitrate: _____. (pp. 396–397)
    1. Caustic
    2. Mydriotic
    3. Carminative
    4. Diuretic

3. Expands or dilates blood vessels: _____. (pp. 396–397)
    1. Vasodilators
    2. Vasoconstrictors
    3. Carminative
    4. Mydriatic

4. Reduces pain, for example, aspirin: _____. (pp. 396–397)
    1. Analgesic
    2. Antiseptic
    3. Caustic
    4. Coagulant

5. Used in treatment of anemia, for example, liver extract: _____. (pp. 396–397)
    1. Antianemic
    2. Antispasmodic
    3. Hypnotic
    4. Diaphoretic

6. Helps raise blood pressure: _____. (pp. 396–397)
    1. Vasodilator
    2. Hypotensive
    3. Hormone
    4. Hypertensive

7. Stimulates elimination of urine, often used with medications prescribed to reduce hypertension, for example, thiomirin: _____. (pp. 396–397)
   1. Stimulant
   2. Expectorant
   3. Sedative
   4. Diuretic

8. Slows down growth of bacteria, but does not kill all of the bacteria, for example, hydrogen peroxide: _____. (pp. 396–397)
   1. Antacid
   2. Antitoxin
   3. Antiseptic
   4. Astringent

9. Used to induce coughing; an agent that increases bronchial secretion and facilitates its expulsion, for example, Robitussin: _____. (pp. 396–397)
   1. Expectorant
   2. Emollient
   3. Cathartic
   4. Carminative

10. Destroys microorganisms in the body, for example, penicillin: _____. (pp. 396–397)
    1. Antacids
    2. Mydriotic
    3. Emollient
    4. Antibiotic

11. Laxatives, purgatives, inducing bowel movements, for example, cascara sagrada: _____. (pp. 396–397)
    1. Antacid
    2. Cathartic
    3. Antispasmodic
    4. Hypotensive

12. Destroys pathogenic organism, for example, zepharin chloride: _____. (pp. 396–397)
    1. Diaphoretic
    2. Antibiotic
    3. Antitoxin
    4. Disinfectant

13. Used to induce perspiration: _____. (pp. 396–397)
    1. Emollient
    2. Miotic
    3. Diaphoretic
    4. Mydriatic

14. Relieves smooth muscle contraction, for example, atropine sulfate: _____. (pp. 396–397)
    1. Antianemic
    2. Anticoagulant
    3. Antidote
    4. Antispasmodic

**15.** Causes the blood vessels to narrow or constrict: _____. (pp. 396–397)
1. Vasodilator
2. Vasoconstrictor
3. Antispasmodic
4. Antacid

**16.** Decreases clotting of the blood: _____. (pp. 396–397)
1. Antitoxin
2. Anticoagulant
3. Antianemic
4. Coagulant

## Abbreviations

**1.** diag. (pp. 397–400)
1. Diagnosis
2. Diagram
3. Down from
4. Diagrammatic

**2.** BMR (pp. 397–400)
1. Basic medicinal regimen
2. Basal metabolic rate
3. Base mass required
4. None of these is correct

**3.** noct. (pp. 397–400)
1. Notch
2. At night
3. Nosocomial
4. Notice

**4.** wh.ch. (pp. 397–400)
1. Whooping cough
2. Whiplash characteristic
3. Whip chalasia
4. Wheelchair

**5.** stat. (pp. 397–400)
1. Stationary
2. Statistic
3. Sustained
4. Immediately

**6.** URI (pp. 397–400)
1. Upper respiratory infection
2. Upper resting indicator
3. Upper resistance indicator
4. Upper reading indicated

**7.** Omn. hor. (pp. 397–400)
1. Each 10 hours
2. Every day
3. Every hour
4. Each night

**8.** gm. (pp. 397–400)
1. Gamma globule
2. Grand mal (epilepsy)
3. Groin
4. Gram

**9.** cf. (pp. 397–400)
1. Compare
2. Confused
3. Confrontational
4. Amount

**10.** NPO (pp. 397–400)
1. Nothing by mouth
2. Nothing post operative
3. Note after (the) operation
4. Noted by operator

**11.** Ad. lib. (pp. 397–400)
1. As much as desired
2. Toward the left
3. Administrative liberty
4. Alternate days

**12.** exam. (pp. 397–400)
1. Example
2. Exaggerated
3. Examination
4. Review

**13.** RBC (pp. 397–400)
1. Resting blood count
2. Red blood count
3. Retinal blastoma corion
4. None of these is correct

**14.** TO (pp. 397–400)
1. Per operator
2. By mouth
3. Telephone order
4. Per observations

**15.** Rx. (pp. 397–400)
1. Rexall
2. Prescription
3. Relaxation
4. Rectally

**16.** spec. (pp. 397–400)
   *1.* Special
   *2.* Specific
   *3.* Speculation
   *4.* Specimen

**17.** ung. (pp. 397–400)
   *1.* Ointment
   *2.* Ungrateful
   *3.* Unguinal
   *4.* Ungulate

**18.** qh (pp. 397–400)
   *1.* Every hour
   *2.* As necessary
   *3.* Upon request
   *4.* Quotient (is) higher

**19.** VO (pp. 397–400)
   *1.* Volume observed
   *2.* Velocity observation
   *3.* Verbal order
   *4.* Vital observation

**20.** BE (pp. 397–400)
   *1.* Barium enema
   *2.* Best estimate
   *3.* Most efficient
   *4.* Bronchial emphysema

**21.** prn (pp. 397–400)
   *1.* As directed
   *2.* As ordered
   *3.* As needed
   *4.* As observed

**22.** tab. (pp. 397–400)
   *1.* (to) tabulate
   *2.* Tablet
   *3.* Total
   *4.* Tabescent

**23.** Disch. (pp. 397–400)
   *1.* Discharge
   *2.* Discontinue
   *3.* Disengage
   *4.* Disease

**24.** Omn. noct. (pp. 397–400)
   *1.* All requirements
   *2.* Omentum
   *3.* Omentitis
   *4.* Every night

**25.** tid (pp. 397–400)
   *1.* Treble in dosage
   *2.* Three times a day
   *3.* Triple in dosage
   *4.* Trigonitis

**26.** quotid (pp. 397–400)
   *1.* Hourly
   *2.* Weekly
   *3.* Daily
   *4.* Quotient

**27.** IV (pp. 397–400)
   *1.* Intravenous
   *2.* Intravital
   *3.* Intraventricular
   *4.* Intravasion

**28.** hs (pp. 397–400)
   *1.* Hospital
   *2.* At bedtime
   *3.* On rising
   *4.* Hyaloserositis

**29.** inf. (pp. 397–400)
   *1.* Infinity
   *2.* Infantilism
   *3.* Infusion
   *4.* Infiltration

**30.** FUO (pp. 397–400)
   *1.* Fracture of unknown origin
   *2.* Fistula of unknown origin
   *3.* Fever of unknown origin
   *4.* Fibrosis of unknown origin

**31.** EEG (pp. 397–400)
   *1.* Electroencephalogram
   *2.* Electrocardiogram
   *3.* Exciting electrode graphics
   *4.* Electrogastrograph

**32.** sol. (pp. 397–400)
   *1.* Solution
   *2.* Solar
   *3.* Sole
   *4.* Sun

**33.** u. (pp. 397–400)
   *1.* Unfit
   *2.* Undo
   *3.* Urgent
   *4.* Unit

**34.** surg. (pp. 397–400)
   *1.* Surrogate
   *2.* Surgery
   *3.* Surgical
   *4.* Susceptible

**35.** lab. (pp. 397–400)
   *1.* Labiograph
   *2.* Labionasal
   *3.* Laboratory
   *4.* Labiogingival

## Prefixes

**1.** a-, an-, for example, anorexia: _____. (pp. 400–403)
   *1.* Without
   *2.* Down from
   *3.* Away from
   *4.* Decreasing

**2.** ad-, for example, additive: _____. (pp. 400–403)
   *1.* Toward, to, at
   *2.* From
   *3.* Away
   *4.* Decreasing

**3.** ambi-, for example, ambilateral: _____. (pp. 400–403)
   *1.* Additional
   *2.* Reducing
   *3.* Confusing
   *4.* Both

**4.** angio-, for example, angiofibrosis: _____. (pp. 400–403)
   *1.* Relating to
   *2.* To a vessel
   *3.* Against
   *4.* Differentiated from

**5.** antero-, for example, anteromedian: _____. (pp. 400–403)
   *1.* In front of
   *2.* Away from
   *3.* Down from
   *4.* Relating to

6. apo-, for example, apocleisis: _____. (pp. 400–403)
   1. Relating to
   2. Many
   3. Up, toward
   4. Away from, off

7. arthro-, for example, arthropathy: _____. (pp. 400–403)
   1. Relation to the legs
   2. Relation to the joints
   3. Relation to the neck
   4. Relation to an arthritic condition

8. bi-, for example, bilateral: _____. (pp. 400–403)
   1. Together
   2. Pertaining to
   3. Good
   4. Two

9. brady-, for example, bradycardia: _____. (pp. 400–403)
   1. Fast
   2. Slow
   3. On the side of
   4. Head

10. carcino-, for example, carcinogen: _____. (pp. 400–403)
    1. Pertaining to additives
    2. Pertaining to poisons
    3. Pertaining to a reduction
    4. Pertaining to cancer

11. cata-, for example, catabolism: _____. (pp. 400–403)
    1. Toward
    2. Downward, against
    3. Deriving from
    4. Within, inner

12. cephalo-, for example, cephalogram: (pp. 400–403)
    1. Neck
    2. Shoulder
    3. Trunk of body
    4. Head

13. chiro-, for example, chiroplasty: _____. (pp. 400–403)
    1. Pertaining to the hand
    2. Pertaining to the neck
    3. Pertaining to the body
    4. Pertaining to the head

14. circum-, for example, circumcorneal: _____. (pp. 400–403)
    1. Under
    2. Beneath
    3. Above
    4. Around

**15.** contra-, for example, contraindicated: _____. (pp. 400–403)
    *1.* Without
    *2.* Around
    *3.* Above
    *4.* Against, opposite

**16.** crano-, for example, craniotomy: _____. (pp. 400–403)
    *1.* Pertaining to the neck
    *2.* Pertaining to the spinal cord
    *3.* Pertaining to the head
    *4.* Pertaining to the lower back

**17.** cyto-, for example, cytolysis: _____. (pp. 400–403)
    *1.* Relation to a cell
    *2.* Relation to life
    *3.* Relation to a limb
    *4.* A cleansing

**18.** derm , for example, dermatitis: (pp. 400–403)
    *1.* Pertaining to the skin
    *2.* Pertaining to the lower intestine
    *3.* Relating to germs
    *4.* Pertaining to the skull

**19.** di-, for example, diarthric: _____. (pp. 400–403)
    *1.* Through
    *2.* A cutting of
    *3.* Within
    *4.* Double, twice

**20.** dys-, for example, dysphasia: _____. (pp. 400–403)
    *1.* Away from
    *2.* Down from
    *3.* Within
    *4.* Painful, difficult

**21.** em-, en-, for example, embolic: _____. (pp. 400–403)
    *1.* In
    *2.* Outside of
    *3.* Around
    *4.* Through

**22.** endo-, for example, endocarditis: _____. (pp. 400–403)
    *1.* Within, inner
    *2.* Exterior to
    *3.* Pertaining to
    *4.* Above

**23.** epi-, for example, epidermatitis: _____. (pp. 400–403)
    *1.* Above, upon, over
    *2.* Below
    *3.* Through
    *4.* Surrounding

**24.** fibro-, for example, fibrocarcinoma: _____. (pp. 400–403)
  *1.* Pertaining to a large mass
  *2.* Pertaining to fiber
  *3.* Pertaining to a softening
  *4.* Pertaining to diluting

**25.** glyco-, for example, glycosuria: _____. (pp. 400–403)
  *1.* Relation to sweetness
  *2.* Relation to the head
  *3.* A diminution or decrease
  *4.* Relation to the stomach

**26.** hema-, hemo-, for example, hemorrhage: _____. (pp. 400–403)
  *1.* Pertaining to the liver
  *2.* Pertaining to the pancreas
  *3.* Pertaining to the ductless glands
  *4.* Pertaining to the blood

**27.** hepato-, for example, hepatitis: _____. (pp. 400–403)
  *1.* Lung
  *2.* Liver
  *3.* Heart
  *4.* Limb

**28.** hydro-, for example, hydrocyst: _____. (pp. 400–403)
  *1.* Lymph
  *2.* Water
  *3.* Bile
  *4.* Any secretion

**29.** hypno-, for example, hypnotherapy: _____. (pp. 400–403)
  *1.* Relating to water
  *2.* Relating to a drainage
  *3.* Relating to sleep
  *4.* Relating to depression

**30.** hystero-, for example, hysterogram: _____. (pp. 400–403)
  *1.* Relating to the blood
  *2.* Relating to the cells
  *3.* Relating to the uterus
  *4.* A cutting out

**31.** infra-, for example, infracardiac: _____. (pp. 400–403)
  *1.* Above
  *2.* Beneath, below
  *3.* Beside of
  *4.* In the direction of

**32.** intra-, for example, intracutaneous: _____. (pp. 400–403)
1. Within
2. On the surface
3. Exterior to
4. Away from

**33.** osteo-, for example, osteoporosis: _____. (pp. 400–403)
1. Pertaining to an opening
2. Pertaining to the bones
3. Pertaining to the body
4. Pertaining to the skull

**34.** pachy-, for example, pachylosis: _____. (pp. 400–403)
1. Thick
2. Thin
3. Scattered
4. Uncoordinated

**35.** para-, for example, paralysis: _____. (pp. 400–403)
1. Between
2. Beneath
3. Instead of
4. Beyond, beside

**36.** per-, for example, perfusion: _____. (pp. 400–403)
1. Through
2. About
3. Down from
4. False

**37.** phlebo- for example, phlebitis: _____. (pp. 400–403)
1. Relating to an artery
2. Relating to phlegm
3. Relating to a vein
4. Relating to a nephron

**38.** poly-, for example, polycardia: _____. (pp. 400–403)
1. Many, much
2. Happiness
3. Depressed
4. Shiny

**39.** pseudo-, for example, pseudodementia: _____. (pp. 400–403)
1. Many
2. Fresh
3. New
4. False

**40.** pyo-, for example, pyoderma: _____. (pp. 400–403)
   *1.* Signifying fire
   *2.* Signifying pus
   *3.* Signifying desire for a change
   *4.* Signifying a deepening

**41.** rhino-, for example, rhinoplasty: _____. (pp. 400–403)
   *1.* A large beast
   *2.* Nose
   *3.* Liver
   *4.* Kidney

**42.** tachy-, for example, tachycardia: _____. (pp. 400–403)
   *1.* Poor taste
   *2.* Rapid
   *3.* Slow
   *4.* Indifferent

**43.** uni-, for example, unicellular: _____. (pp. 400–403)
   *1.* All
   *2.* Neither
   *3.* One
   *4.* Many

**44.** intro-, for example, introgastric: _____. (pp. 400–403)
   *1.* In, into
   *2.* On the outside of
   *3.* Surrounding
   *4.* Below

**45.** labio-, for example, labiocervical: _____. (pp. 400–403)
   *1.* Relating to the lip
   *2.* Relating to nearby tissues
   *3.* Surrounding
   *4.* Containing

**46.** mega-, for example, megacardia: _____. (pp. 400–403)
   *1.* Large, oversize
   *2.* Relating to the intestines
   *3.* Relating to the meninges
   *4.* Relating to the brain

**47.** myo-, for example, myocardial infarction: _____. (pp. 400–403)
   *1.* Relating to an enlargement
   *2.* Relating to a metastasis
   *3.* Relating to muscle
   *4.* Relating to nerve fibers

**48.** necro-, for example, necrosis: _____. (pp. 400–403)
   *1.* Darkening
   *2.* Death
   *3.* Enlargement
   *4.* Shrinkage

**49.** omo-, for example, omodynia: _____. (pp. 400–403)
   *1.* Pertaining to the knee joint
   *2.* Pertaining to the shoulder
   *3.* A reduction
   *4.* An unexplained enlargement

**50.** odont-, for example, odontalgia: _____. (pp. 400–403)
   *1.* Relating to the teeth
   *2.* Relating to the upper back
   *3.* Relating to the spine
   *4.* Relating to an opening

## Suffixes

**1.** -ac, for example, cardiac: _____. (pp. 404–405)
   *1.* Flowing from
   *2.* Following
   *3.* Pertaining to
   *4.* Underneath

**2.** -algia, for example, neuralgia: _____. (pp. 404–405)
   *1.* Heat
   *2.* A loss of
   *3.* Pleasure
   *4.* Pain

**3.** -centesis, for example, paracentesis: _____. (pp. 404–405)
   *1.* Centered
   *2.* One-sided
   *3.* Occurring on both sides
   *4.* Surgical puncture

**4.** -clysis, for example, enteroclysis: _____. (pp. 404–405)
   *1.* Controlling
   *2.* Reducing infection of
   *3.* Excision of
   *4.* Washing, irrigation

**5.** -cyle, for example, hematocyle: _____. (pp. 404–405)
   *1.* Organ
   *2.* Tissue
   *3.* Cell
   *4.* Appendage

**6.** -emesis, for example, hyperemesis: _____. (pp. 404–405)
   *1.* Cleansing
   *2.* Vomiting
   *3.* Coughing
   *4.* Shrinking

7. -genesis, for example, carcinogenesis: _____. (pp. 404–405)
   1. Condition of reducing
   2. Reshaping
   3. Reducing
   4. Condition of producing

8. -lith, for example, nephrolith: _____. (pp. 404–405)
   1. Graph
   2. Chart
   3. Figure
   4. Stone

9. -malacia, for example, osteomalacia: _____. (pp. 404–405)
   1. Hardening
   2. Softening
   3. Swelling
   4. Suture

10. -odynia, for example, cardiodynia: _____. (pp. 404–405)
    1. A painful condition
    2. An improving condition
    3. A reduction in
    4. Reduction in size of

11. -opsy, for example, biopsy: _____. (pp. 404–405)
    1. To view
    2. To reduce in size
    3. To excise
    4. To cut

12. -orrhaphy, for example, gastrorrhaphy: _____. (pp. 404–405)
    1. Appetite, desire
    2. Deficiency
    3. To view
    4. Suture

13. -orrhea, for example, gastrorrhea: _____. (pp. 404–405)
    1. FLow, discharge
    2. To view
    3. Incision
    4. Fixation

14. -otomy, for example, nephrotomy: _____. (pp. 404–405)
    1. To remove
    2. Incision, to cut into
    3. A state of
    4. A poor prognosis

15. -penia, for example, leukopenia: _____. (pp. 404–405)
    1. Excess
    2. Deficiency
    3. Discharge
    4. Tumor

**16.** -pexy, for example, nephropexy: _____. (pp. 404–405)
1. Disruption
2. Discharge
3. Seepage
4. Fixation, to put into place

**17.** -phasia, for example, aphasia: _____. (pp. 404–405)
1. Spasm
2. Hardening
3. Softening
4. Speech

**18.** -phobia, for example, claustrophobia: _____. (pp. 404–405)
1. Enjoyment
2. Contentment
3. Fear
4. Speech

**19.** -rhythmia, for example, arrhythmia: _____. (pp. 404–405)
1. Rhythmic
2. Rheumatoid
3. Irregular
4. Variegated

**20.** -spasm, for example, myospasm: _____. (pp. 404–405)
1. Sudden violent involuntary contraction of muscles
2. Sudden violent voluntary contraction of muscles
3. Outburst
4. Hemorrhage

**21.** -stenosis, for example, arteriostenosis: _____. (pp. 404–405)
1. Widening
2. Tightening, stricture
3. Relaxation
4. Spasm

**22.** -tripsy, for example, lithotripsy: _____. (pp. 404–405)
1. A closing
2. A widening
3. A crushing
4. A reduction

**23.** -uria, for example, albuminuria: _____. (pp. 404–405)
1. Stone
2. Urine
3. Reduction
4. Enlargement

## THE AGING PROCESS AS IT RELATES TO DISEASES COMMON TO THE NURSING HOME POPULATION

1.  The bones, muscles, cartilage, tendons, and joints use in movement are: _____. (p. 406)
    1. The nervous system
    2. Respiration
    3. The reproductive system
    4. The musculoskeletal system

2.  The system that circulates blood is also called the _____. (p. 406)
    1. Gastric system
    2. Defense system
    3. Cardiovascular system
    4. The nervous system

3.  When the health of cells has deteriorated it usually is due to a decrease in effectiveness of the _____, interfering with the supply of nutrients to them. (p. 406)
    1. Cardiovascular system
    2. Nervous system
    3. Musculoskeletal system
    4. Regenerative capacities

4.  A stroke occurs when the lack of oxygen to an area of the brain causes _____. (p. 411)
    1. Insomnia
    2. Increased olfactory acuity
    3. Ductless gland system
    4. Permanent damage

5.  An elderly person whose blood pressure is consistently greater than 160/95 is considered to have _____. (p. 410)
    1. Hypertension
    2. A severe stroke
    3. A strong heart
    4. Low blood pressure

6.  The left side of the brain controls the functions on the _____ side of the body. (p. 423)
    1. Distal
    2. Front
    3. Left
    4. Right

7.  A disease resulting from loss of elasticity in the lung tissues causing carbon dioxide to build up is _____. (p. 418)
    1. Kidney failure
    2. Emphysema
    3. Lung cancer
    4. Pneumonia

8. A progressive disease for which there is no cure, characterized by tremor, rigidity, or muscle stiffness and bradykinesia is _____. (p. 427)
   1. Diverticulitis
   2. Parkinson's disease
   3. Delirium tremens
   4. Chrone's disease

9. Difficulty in swallowing or transferring food from the mouth to the esophagus is called _____. (p. 441)
   1. Esophagitis
   2. Dysphagia
   3. Peptic ulcer
   4. Hiatal hernia

10. The transformation process in which nutrients undergo various chemical reactions is _____. (p. 443)
   1. Dysphagia
   2. Diet
   3. Metabolism
   4. Caloric intake

11. Plasma, which carries red blood cells, and lymph, which carries white blood cells, are examples of _____. (p. 444)
   1. Metabolism
   2. Carbohydrates
   3. Body fluids
   4. Liquids

12. Measuring daily fasting blood sugar level and measuring the amount of glucose in the urine are tests used in the treatment of _____. (p. 447)
   1. Diabetes
   2. Acute vitamin deficiencies
   3. Hodgkin's disease
   4. Rheumatic heart disease

13. Infections associated with institutionalization are referred to as _____ infections. (p. 449)
   1. Nosocomial
   2. Internal
   3. Benign
   4. Unnecessary

14. Decubitus ulcers, once formed, can _____. (p. 451)
   1. Increase longevity
   2. Become infected and form cavities of dead tissue
   3. Benefit the various organs in the body
   4. Stimulate resident activity

15. The leading types of cancer among males seen in the nursing facility are cancer of the _____. (p. 456)
   1. Lung and brain
   2. Prostate gland and rectum
   3. Brain and colon
   4. Lung, colon, and rectum

**16.** Falls among persons over 65 years of age account for more than ____% of deaths that result from all falls. (p. 460)
1. 30
2. 70
3. 95
4. 40

**17.** Chronic renal failure that has progressed to the stage where little or no urine is being produced is called _____. (p. 464)
1. Kidney failure
2. End-stage renal disease
3. Renal deficiency
4. Renal keratosis

**18.** A study by Stilwell and O'Conner indicated that among persons studied _____. (p. 471)
1. Older people remain interested in sex
2. Older people find each other attractive
3. All of these were findings in the Stilwell and O'Conner study
4. Sexuality contributes to overall well-being

**19.** The line between disabling mental illnesses and the day to day effects of coping with old age _____. (p. 473)
1. Can be readily identified
2. Is often blurred
3. Can be measured
4. Is usually available on the nursing reports

**20.** In the nursing facility, person-centered administration means focusing on _____. (p. 475)
1. Excellence in pain management
2. The quality of resident life
3. Excellence in medication administration
4. Keeping staff trained

**21.** The process by which the body breaks down the foods eaten into a form usable by individual cells is _____. (p. 438)
1. Digestion
2. Dieting
3. Processing
4. Metabolism

**22.** Combined with oxygen, nutrients permit individual cells to perform chemical reactions that _____. (p. 407)
1. Destroy vitamins
2. Produce energy
3. Stop chemical reactions
4. Facilitate chemical reactions

**23.** Peripheral vascular disease commonly refers to the increased resistance in the blood vessels _____. (p. 412)
1. Primarily in the head
2. In the chest region
3. Crohn's disease
4. In the extremities

**24.** When the heart muscle itself suffers from a lack of oxygen due to blockages in the arteries that usually supply it, it is known as _____. (p. 412)
   1. Coronary artery disease
   2. Decreased blood flow
   3. Decreased blood supply
   4. Progressive organ failure

**25.** Blood being backed up in the circulatory system causing fluids to leak out of the bloodstream is symptomatic of _____. (p. 414)
   1. Risk of heart attack
   2. Anorexia
   3. Congestive heart failure
   4. An aging resident with kidney infection

**26.** Because tuberculosis can be transmitted through secretions or when a resident coughs, it is considered _____. (p. 421)
   1. An old person's disease
   2. The onset of MRSA
   3. An infectious disease
   4. A lung disease

**27.** The primary problem resulting in glaucoma is _____. (p. 424)
   1. Pressure due to failure of fluids to drain normally
   2. Reduction in the level of aqueous humor
   3. Changes in the retina
   4. Shrinkage of the lens of the eye

**28.** The digestive system is referred to as the alimentary tract or the _____. (p. 439)
   1. The digestive tract
   2. Upper and lower intestine
   3. Bowels
   4. Gastrointestinal tract

**29.** Sharp burning abdominal pain 1–4 hours after eating, nausea, weight loss, and blood in stools can be symptoms of _____. (p. 442)
   1. Increased risk of stroke
   2. Fats
   3. Excessive protein
   4. An ulcer

**30.** Carbohydrates can be broken down readily into fuel for the body. Two common sources are _____. (p. 444)
   1. Starches and sugars
   2. Minerals and vitamins
   3. Sodium and its substitutes
   4. Calcium and iron

**31.** During the years 1993–2008, the percent of residents in U.S. nursing facilities who had psychological diagnoses _____. (p. 430)
   1. Increased to 47% up from 37%
   2. Remained steady
   3. Declined
   4. Rose, then fell back

**32.** Gastrostomy tubes for residents needing long-term tube feeding may be preferred over nasogastric tubes because there is no chance that fluids may be _____. (p. 445)
1. Leaked
2. Over controlled
3. Lost
4. Aspirated

**33.** Diabetes occurs when the body is unable to metabolize _____ because of a problem with a hormone called insulin. (p. 446)
1. Vitamins
2. Minerals
3. Glucose
4. Potassium

**34.** Anemia occurs when there is a difficulty with the _____ blood cells, resulting in the body not getting enough oxygen. (p. 446)
1. White
2. Red
3. White and red
4. Disease fighting

**35.** The skin, the acid composition of gastric juices, and the urine are _____ that help protect the body. (p. 448)
1. Barrier-type defenses
2. Ineffective-type defenses
3. Immune defenses
4. Internal organs

**36.** Whenever foreign material or _____ enter the body, the components of the immune system recognize this and mobilize for an attack response. (p. 448)
1. Antighesis
2. Antigens
3. Antidotes
4. Antibacterial

**37.** Redness surrounding areas of skin that may become infected is called the _____ response. (p. 449)
1. Action
2. Antiallergic
3. Offense
4. Inflammation

**38.** The tough, dry, wrinkled skin sometimes observed among elderly persons may work to _____ the barrier effect of the skin. (p. 450)
1. Improve
2. Diminish
3. Rejuvenate
4. Heighten

**39.** The formation of a skin ulcer can occur when _____. (p. 452)
1. The body's chemical defense mechanism suddenly degrades
2. The weight of the body exerts unusual pressure on internal soft tissue
3. Patients reach advanced age
4. Patients' diets are altered

**40.** Residents most at risk of developing pressure sores are those _____. (p. 452)
1. With poor personal hygiene
2. With excessive fat tissue
3. Who have poor dentition
4. Who are immobile

**41.** The percentage of U.S. nursing home residents who were chairbound in 2008 was just over (p. 453)
1. 95%
2. 10%
3. 25%
4. 50%

**42.** Hypothermia is often difficult to diagnose because symptoms may be similar to _____. (p. 455)
1. Mild anorexia
2. A minor stroke
3. A massive heart attack
4. Advanced cancer symptoms

**43.** The proportion of residents in U.S. nursing facilities during 1993–2008 who received special skin care _____. (p. 454)
1. Nearly doubled
2. Remained the same
3. Decreased
4. Increased fourfold

**44.** Joints are the points in the body at which _____. (p. 457-458)
1. Bones are always fused
2. The ends of two bones meet
3. Breaks have earlier occurred
4. Ulcers form

**45.** There is some consensus among researchers that during the aging process the total amount of bone in the body _____. (p. 458)
1. Decreases
2. Increases
3. Becomes elevated
4. Remains stable

**46.** The proportion of residents in U.S. nursing homes during 1993–2008 who were incontinent remained about _____. (p. 465)
1. More than 90%
2. Too few to meaningfully measure
3. 10%
4. 50%

**47.** Orthostatic hypotension is _____. (p. 395)
1. Decreased blood pressure on standing
2. Excessive irritability
3. Decreased irritability
4. Degenerative bone disease leading to weakening of the bones

**48.** In addition to removing waste materials from the blood stream, the kidneys also help regulate the _____. (p. 462)
1. Amount of body fluids
2. Ductless gland system
3. Pituitary gland
4. Thalamus gland

**49.** Itchy and dry skin, mental confusion, weakness, muscle cramps, nausea, vomiting, and diarrhea can all be symptoms of _____. (p. 464)
1. Oncoming chronic renal failure
2. Hyperactive kidneys
3. Excessive rate of urine production
4. Constant urine production

**50.** Patients unable to urinate can be _____ periodically following fluid intake. (p. 466)
1. Advised
2. Ambulated
3. Catheterized
4. Rejoined

**51.** During midlife women experience cessation of egg production, and hence of menstruation, called _____. (p. 468)
1. Menopause
2. Hysterectomy
3. Genital prolapse
4. Prostatitis

**52.** An elderly male nursing facility resident with painful urination and blood in the urine should be checked for _____. (p. 469)
1. Rectal cancer
2. Dermal cancer
3. Prostatitis
4. Dysphagia

**53.** The incidence of heart attack or stroke during sexual intercourse _____. (p. 470)
1. Is a major concern for nursing home physicians
2. Has been identified as a valid health issue
3. Is very low
4. Has been declining during the past decade

**54.** Fantasizing, avoidance of eye contact, fidgeting, insomnia, isolation from others, and hostile or dependent behaviors are thought to be manifestations of _____. (p. 471)
1. Personal abilities
2. Repressive staff
3. Anxiety
4. Exploratory behavior

**55.** Psychotropic drugs exert an effect primarily on the _____. (p. 472)
1. Brain
2. Digits
3. Internal organs
4. Extremities

**56.** Nearly _____ of all residents in U.S. nursing homes in 2008 were receiving psychoactive drugs. (pp. 472–473)
1. 10%
2. A quarter
3. Three fourths
4. Two-thirds

**57.** There are losses incoming residents inevitably experience, and _____. (p. 387)
1. These can never be understood
2. They are most difficult to identify
3. There are also gains
4. They are quickly forgotten

**58.** Anger and anxiety typically associated with being admitted to a nursing facility can lead to _____. (p. 473)
1. An easy adjustment
2. Admission-associated depression
3. Hyperactivity
4. Relief

**59.** The number of facilities receiving citations for improper restraint use in 2008 was about_____ than in 1993. (p. 475)
1. 5% less
2. One-third less
3. Out of proportion
4. Dramatically more

**60.** Experience suggests that it is important to identify a depression on top of _____. (p. 475)
1. Dementia
2. Advanced psychosis
3. Early Alzheimer's
4. Advanced Alzheimer's

# 6

# Facility Policies

# Putting the System Together

In Part 6, answers can be found in *Nursing Home Administration*, Sixth Edition and *Nursing Home Federal Requirements: Guidelines to Surveyors and Survey Protocols*, 7th Edition, by James E. Allen, MSPH, PhD, CNHA (Springer Publishing Company). Those found in *Nursing Home Federal Requirements* are distinguished by the reference (see Federal Requirements).

# 6.1

# Setting Policies for the Facility

## 6.1.1 ADMINISTRATION POLICIES

1. If a nursing facility has been certified by Medicare and Medicaid under Final Rules and federal requirements, in effect, it _____. (see Federal Requirements App. P and PP) (p. 482)
   1. Can be exempted from state and local licensure requirements
   2. Must still meet all state and local licensure requirements
   3. Is deemed to have met all state and local licensure requirements
   4. May apply for a waiver from state requirements

2. Establishing and implementing policies regarding the management of the facility is assigned to _____. (see Federal Requirements App. P and PP) (p. 482)
   1. The administrator
   2. The owner(s)
   3. The governing body or persons designated as such
   4. The facility staff

3. In order to begin collecting better data about the nursing home industry, federal legislation mandated development and use of _____. (see Federal Requirements App. P and PP) (p. 523)
   1. The Comprehensive Care Approach
   2. A Minimum Data Set
   3. Changes in record keeping
   4. A state-developed data collection

4. The comprehensive care plan does not include a/an _____. (see Federal Requirements App. P and PP) (p. 506)
   1. Attending physician
   2. Registered nurse caregiver
   3. Resident
   4. Medical director

5. If a nursing facility has been certified by Medicare and Medicaid under Final Rules and federal requirements, in effect, it _____. (see Federal Requirements App. P and PP (p. 482)
   1. Can be exempted from state and local licensure requirements
   2. Must still meet all state and local licensure requirements
   3. Is deemed to have met all state and local licensure requirements
   4. May apply for a waiver from state requirements

6. Establishing and implementing policies regarding the management of the facility is assigned to _____. (see Federal Requirements App. P and PP) (p. 482)
   1. The administrator
   2. The owner(s)
   3. The governing body or persons designated as such
   4. The facility staff

7. Nurse aides who have completed a training and competency evaluation program and passed the required competency test(s) _____. (see Federal Requirements App. P and PP) (p. 484)
   1. May serve at any facility
   2. Must still be judged by surveyors as competent to provide services
   3. May, at their option, be registered with the state nurses aide registry
   4. May sit for training for nurses aide assistant, IV

8. Responsibility for ascertaining professional performance standards for licensed, certified, or registered allied health persons used by the facility rests with the _____. (see Federal Requirements App. P and PP) (p. 482)
   1. Respective certifying or registering boards
   2. Resident or her responsible party
   3. State
   4. Facility

9. Organizations that actually pay the Medicare claims submitted by doctors and other medical suppliers are called _____. (see Federal Requirements App. P and PP) (p. 497)
   1. Carriers
   2. Medicare contractors
   3. Third-party payers
   4. Intermediaries

## Resource Utilization

**10.** The facility is not required to use its resource effectively and efficiently to attain highest practical _____. (p. 481)
   *1.* Resident physical well being
   *2.* Resident mental well being
   *3.* Profitability
   *4.* Resident psychosocial wellbeing

## Mental Illness

**11.** A person who is determined by the state mental health authority to need nursing facility service but is receiving active treatment for mental illness _____. (see Federal Requirements App. P and PP) (pp. 485–486)
   *1.* Can be admitted
   *2.* Must not be admitted
   *3.* May be admitted if medical director authorizes it
   *4.* Must go to the state mental hospital or equivalent

**12.** Each facility must designate a physician to serve as medical director _____. (see Federal Requirements App. P and PP) (p. 485)
   *1.* On a part-time basis
   *2.* On a full-time basis
   *3.* On a part- or full-time basis
   *4.* When needed

## Compliance with Laws

**13.** The administrator believes that once his obligation to meet federal state and local laws is metl he has satisfied the requirements applicable to the operation of his facility. The administrator is _____. (pp. 481–482)
   *1.* Following all requirements
   *2.* By definition meeting standards
   *3.* Exceeding minimum operational standards
   *4.* Only partially correct

**14.** The terms for Medicare and Medicaid participating homes used in the Final Rules effect are _____. (see Federal Requirements App. P and PP) (p. 482)
   *1.* Nursing home and nursing facility
   *2.* Medicaid facility and Medicare facility
   *3.* Skilled nursing facility and nursing facility
   *4.* Approved facility and licensed facility

**15.** Having a transfer agreement with one or more hospitals is _____. (see Federal Requirements App. P and PP) (p. 482)
   *1.* Good practice
   *2.* A risk management measure
   *3.* A condition of participation requirement
   *4.* Wise step-in preparation for emergency situations

**16.** Nursing homes are licensed by _____. (see Federal Requirements App. P and PP) (pp. 481–482)
1. The counties
2. The states
3. The federal regional government arms
4. Centers for Medicare and Medicaid

**17.** Regulations such as those implementing Medicare and Medicaid; Requirements for Long-term Care Facilities, are first published in the _____. (see Federal Requirements App. P and PP) (p. 483)
1. U.S. Code
2. National Register
3. Congressional Record
4. Federal Register

## Governing Body

**18.** All facilities are required to _____. (p. 482)
1. Have a governing body
2. Have an adequately functioning administrator who reports to a corporate board
3. Have a governing body or designated persons
4. Have a governing body or designated persons functioning as a governing body

## Transfer Agreement

**19.** The facility administrator establishes written transfer agreements with two local hospitals, one of which is approved only for participation under the Medicare program, and the second approved only for participation under Medicaid. The administrator has _____. (p. 482)
1. Failed to meet transfer agreement requirements
2. Accomplished the minimum required by the Federal Regulations
3. More that met the minimum required—an agreement with one of these hospitals would meet requirements
4. Assured that needed transfers can be accomplished

**20.** The transfer agreements signed by the administrator assure that the Medical and other information needed for care and treatment of residents, and guarantees that a bed will be available for the resident upon his return from the hospital. This is the entire agreement. A visiting surveyor would _____. (p. 482)
1. Find this acceptable
2. Require changes to the transfer agreement
3. Believe residents of that facility were being adequately protected
4. Feel comfortable that a resident's right to return to the facility has been protected

**21.** The discharge social worker at the hospital determines that the resident cared for under the transfer agreement should return, not to the facility, but be placed in an assisted living facility that is a less expensive setting. Normally, _____. (p. 482)
1. This is inappropriate
2. This is appropriate
3. This is outside the prerogative of a hospital
4. This frowned upon by Medicare

## Changes in Ownership

**22.** If persons with controlling interest in the facility, the company owning the facility or the administrator or director of nursing change, the facility should _____. (p. 482)
1. Call and inform the state facility licensing agency
2. Inform the state licensing agency in writing
3. Inform the Medicare Intermediary
4. Inform the state Medicaid officials

## 6.1.2 FACILITY PERSONNEL POLICIES

## Activities Program Professional

**23.** The administrator decides the trained therapeutic recreation specialist is too costly for the facility and hires instead a less expensive qualified occupational therapy assistant. This is _____. (p. 483)
1. Within the federal hiring guidelines
2. Outside the federal hiring guidelines
3. An unfortunate decision
4. Likely to not be a cost effective decision

## Social Services

**24.** The recently graduated social worker job applicant for a 140-bed facility states she has a bachelor's degree in psychology and one year's experience as supervisor of four social workers at a nearby nursing hospital. The administrator should _____. (p. 483)
1. Be satisfied that the applicant meets requirements for his facility
2. Hire the applicant
3. Explore the applicant's experience in more depth
4. Be pleased that the applicant has supervised four social workers

## Registered Nurse

**25.** The administrator of a 50-bed facility asks the director of nursing to serve as both director of nursing and as a charge nurse on the weekend shift. (p. 483)
1. This is appropriate
2. Minimum staffing has been met
3. Minimum staffing has not been met
4. Not permitted

**26.** If a facility provides the stated minimum number of hours per resident day of care, a state or federal inspector _____. (see Federal Requirements App. P and PP) (p. 483)
1. May still cite nursing for insufficient staffing
2. Will pass the facility on staffing
3. Will require the facility to maintain that ratio
4. May, at her discretion, reduce the staffing required

27. If the administrator of an average daily total occupancy of 80 residents requires the director of nursing to serve as charge nurse, the administrator _____. (see Federal Requirements App. P and PP) (p. 483)
    1. Has met Final Rules requirements
    2. Needs to routinely report the assignment to the State
    3. Has failed to meet Final Rules requirements
    4. Has exceeded Final Rules requirements

## Consultant Pharmacist

28. The consultant pharmacist at his monthly visit requires the director of nursing to provide to him a reconciliation report for all controlled drugs signed verified by the director of nursing. The pharmacist _____. (p. 483)
    1. Has met his obligations
    2. Has acted in good faith
    3. Should determine himself that drug records are in order
    4. Is meeting the expectations of Medicare and Medicaid record keeping

## Nurse Aides

29. The personnel director recommends a part-time nurses aide who has worked at the facility for the past six months and is nearing the end of her competency evaluation program. The administrator should feel that the personnel director is _____. (p. 484)
    1. Doing a good job
    2. Not understanding the requirements
    3. Smart to have a person under observation for six months before permanent hiring
    4. Functioning quite well

## In-Service Education of Nurse Aides

30. At least every 12 months the facility requires all full- and part-time nurses aide to fill in a report on his/her continuing education done by each aide in the facility. This report is then filed in the employee's personnel file. The facility is _____. (p. 484)
    1. Meeting reporting requirements
    2. Right to keep the signed report in the employee's personnel file
    3. Not keeping adequate records of training
    4. Failing to train based on outcome of these reviews

## Use of Outside Resources

31. When the facility does not employ a qualified professional to furnish a service to be provided by the facility, the facility _____. (p. 484)
    1. Can provide a list of suitably qualified professionals in the community
    2. Can seek volunteer help for unmet services
    3. Must use the local hospital
    4. Must have that service furnished

### Disaster and Emergency Preparedness

32. The facility should train all employees in emergency procedures _____. (p. 484)
    1. By the end of the first week on the job
    2. The first day on the job
    3. As soon as training staff are available
    4. Before the employee's first day on the job

33. The facility must train _____ in emergency procedures _____. (p. 484)
    1. All caregiver employees/when they begin to work
    2. All employees/when they begin to work
    3. Designated employees/within three weeks of employment
    4. New employees/within one week

### Not Employ Certain Individuals

34. When a facility learns a court of law has taken action against one of its employees, indicating unfitness for service, the facility must _____. (pp. 484–485)
    1. Fire that employee immediately
    2. Give the employee two weeks' notice
    3. Require additional inservice education for that employee
    4. Report the court's action to licensing authorities

35. Ms. Brown alleges for the twelfth documented time that she was abused by an employee. The facility _____. (pp. 484–485)
    1. Is justified in documenting, but not investigating the matter
    2. Should perform the thirteenth investigation
    3. Should report the alleged complaint to the state
    4. Should consider transferring that resident to a more suitable facility

## 6.1.3 DIETARY

36. If the facility does not employ a fulltime qualified dietitian, the facility _____. (p. 485)
    1. Can appoint instead a full time director of food services
    2. May seek consultation from the outside
    3. Designates a director of food services who receives consultation from a qualified dietitian
    4. Employs a nutrition expert who advises the director of food service

37. The facility must employ a _____ either full-time, part-time, or on a consultant basis. (see Federal Requirements App. P and PP) (p. 485)
    1. Director of food services
    2. Chef
    3. Sufficient dietary staff
    4. Qualified dietitian

## 6.1.4  ADMISSIONS POLICIES

**38.** Orders for routine care or to improve the resident's functional abilities must be available _____. (pp. 485–486)
   *1.* At admission
   *2.* Within 24 hours of admission
   *3.* Within 36 hours of admission
   *4.* By the second shift after readmission

## 6.1.6  REHABILITATION POLICIES

**39.** If mental health rehabilitative services for mental illness or mental retardation are required in the resident's plan of care, the facility _____. (p. 486)
   *1.* May seek to transfer the resident to a mental health services setting
   *2.* Must transfer the resident to a mental health services setting
   *3.* Must provide such services in house
   *4.* Must provide in house or obtain such services

**40.** The care plan team determines that, although they had not anticipated it, the resident needs physical therapy. The facility should _____. (p. 486)
   *1.* Assign the therapy to a qualified physical therapist either in house or from outside
   *2.* Get a physician's written order
   *3.* Get authorization from the Medicare provider
   *4.* Begin the physical therapy as soon as possible

## 6.1.7  RESIDENT RIGHTS

### Incompetence/Competence
**41.** A resident who has been determined by the courts to be incompetent decides he no longer wants the court appointed representative to handle his personal funds and asks the facility to establish a personal funds account for him. The facility should_____. (p. 491)
   *1.* Establish a personal funds account for that resident
   *2.* Seek the advice of an attorney
   *3.* Ask the court appointed representative for permission to establish an account
   *4.* Get the advice of the facility accountant

**42.** Perhaps the most basic purpose of the new management of personal resident funds rules is to _____. (see Federal Requirements App. P and PP) (p. 491)
   *1.* Reduce resident confusion about finances
   *2.* Improve facility accounting efficiency
   *3.* Improve interest rates to residents by pooling resident funds
   *4.* Avoid commingling resident funds with facility funds

**43.** Notifying _____ residents when their account reaches _____ less than the _____ resource limit for one person is required. (see Federal Requirements App. P and PP) (p. 491)
1. Medicare/$200/SSI
2. Medicaid/$300/SSA
3. Medicaid/$200/SSI
4. All/$200/personal funds

**44.** Upon discovering that the new intake social worker required the individual holding durable power of attorney for the patient's funds to sign a contract guaranteeing payment from that patient's funds, the administrator should _____. (see Federal Requirements App. P and PP) (p.489)
1. Discourage the social worker from finding similar admissions
2. Revoke the guarantee of payment document
3. Discipline the social worker
4. Praise the intake social worker

**45.** Rights of residents who are adjudged incompetent by a court are exercised by _____. (see Federal Requirements App. P and PP) (p. 487)
1. The locally appointed ombudsman
2. The family
3. A person appointed by the court
4. The responsible adult

**46.** Under the Final Rules, right to immediate access to any resident by representatives of the State, ombudsman, protection agencies, and advocacy agencies is _____. (see Federal Requirements App. P and PP) (p. 494)
1. Subject to resident approval
2. Unrestricted
3. Carefully set out as to time and place
4. Subject to facility approval

**47.** A representative of the state ombudsman office demands to see the clinical record of a Medicaid resident who had written he wanted no one to have access to his clinical record. Upon receiving the request, you, the administrator, should _____. (see Federal Requirements App. P and PP) (p. 494)
1. Deny permission to the ombudsman
2. Provide access to the record requested by the ombudsman
3. Tell the ombudsman you will seek legal counsel, then respond
4. Ask the ombudsman to return at a later time

## Rights Without Reprisal

**48.** The resident hangs a religious ornament above his bed. Several nurse aides are offended and feel it is inappropriate. The facility administrator should _____. (p. 487)
1. Seek a resident council opinion
2. Advise the aides that this is appropriate
3. Try to enforce the separation of church and state rules
4. Get the facility attorney involved

## Resident Rights to Records

**49.** A resident may refuse to release personal and clinical records when _____. (see Federal Requirements App. P and PP) (p. 488)
  1. Transferred to another health care facility
  2. Third-party payment contracts seek it
  3. Required by law
  4. Required by the duly appointed state ombudsman

**50.** A resident asks the afternoon nurse on duty to access his patient records. The nurse responds that she will have the records made available by late tomorrow morning. The nurse's response is _____. (p. 488)
  1. A denial of resident rights
  2. Appropriate
  3. An unpermitted delay
  4. Clearly a delaying tactic

**51.** Congress intends that residents have the right to inspect, upon 48 hours notice, _____. (see Federal Requirements App. P and PP) (p. 488)
  1. Their medical record
  2. The plan of care
  3. Medication records
  4. All their records

## Resident Rights to Health Status Information

**52.** A resident is concerned about her cognitive status and asks to see all the facility has in her records about her cognitive status, including tests administered at admission four weeks earlier. The resident is _____. (p. 488)
  1. Unnecessarily worried
  2. Inappropriate
  3. Asking for information the facility should withhold
  4. Within her rights

**53.** The new resident speaks only Japanese. Before the resident was admitted, the facility advised her through her interpreter that no one in the facility spoke Japanese and that solely sign language would be used. Upon examining this admission condition in the resident's records, the surveyor would _____. (p. 489)
  1. Feel the facility had made a reasonable choice
  2. Ask to see the signage to assess its adequacy
  3. Cite the facility
  4. Suggest ways the facility might better communicate with this resident

## Rights to Advance Directives, to Refuse Treatment or Research

**54.** After the first of 10 scheduled physical therapy sessions following his surgery, the resident tells the physical therapist he is not going to keep the final 9 appointments. The resident is _____. (p. 489)
  1. Making a foolish decision
  2. Exceeding his rights to control his health care
  3. Within his rights
  4. Making a questionable decision

**55.** The resident decides to discontinue all the 9 drugs being administered daily. The facility staff feel this may result in a coma likely followed by death. The facility _____. (p. 489)
1. Can modify this decision as needed to keep the resident alive
2. Must comply and maintain resident at highest level within that decision
3. Must contact and follow the physician's orders
4. Should consider transferring the resident

**56.** Informing a resident of his rights is required _____. (p. 488)
1. Within 24 hours of admission
2. Prior to admission
3. Prior to or at admission
4. As a courtesy to each entering resident

## Work

**57.** A resident may perform services for the facility if the services are _____.(see Federal Requirements App. P and PP) (pp. 493–494)
1. Voluntary
2. Paid at or above prevailing rates
3. In the plan of care
4. Light duty in nature

**58.** When the physician decides to discontinue an existing form of treatment due to adverse consequences, the facility _____. (p. 491)
1. Must note this in the resident's care plan
2. Must notify the resident and the resident's representative
3. Inform the pharmacy of this new information
4. Order new replacement drugs

## Protection of Resident Funds

**59.** The facility staff suspect family members are abusing a resident's funds and requires that for the resident's protection his funds must be deposited with the facility. This is _____. (p. 491)
1. A prudent step for the facility
2. Not permitted
3. Subject to review by the owners
4. A routine protection afforded residents by most facilities

**60.** A resident routinely maintained $40. in his personal funds account and is upset to learn the facility has his funds in a non-interest-bearing account. Placing this resident's funds in a non-interest bearing account is _____. (p. 491)
1. Permitted
2. Required
3. Optional if the resident agrees
4. Expected financial behavior

**61.** A facility that informs each resident who is entitled to Medicaid benefits, in writing, at admission and when changes occur of services which are paid for under the State plan has _____. (see Federal Requirements App. P and PP) (p. 491)
1. Met its obligations
2. Exceeded its required information
3. Not fully met its notice of service obligations
4. Properly interpreted the Final Rules requirement to inform

**62.** Upon the death of a Medicaid resident, the facility conveyed the resident's funds within 14 days and promised to forward a final accounting in three weeks. This is _____. (p. 491)
1. Within the required notification periods
2. A failure to meet notification requirements
3. Faster refunding and accounting than required
4. Meeting minimum standards

**63.** As part of a larger chain, the local facility believes that self-insurance plus use of Federal Deposit Insurance Corporation insured accounts is a reasonable protection of resident funds. The surveyor is likely _____. (p. 492)
1. To agree
2. To want to assure financial stability by reviewing the balance sheets for the facility
3. To issue a deficiency
4. Examine the facility's financial track record

## Allowable Charges

**64.** The facility routinely charges all cosmetic and grooming items and services for private, Medicare and Medicaid residents. This charging policy _____. (p. 492)
1. Is permitted at facility discretion
2. Meets Medicare rules, but not Medicaid rules
3. Meets all rules
4. Is not permitted for Medicare and Medicaid residents

**65.** The facility proudly installed flat screen TVs in all resident rooms and added a small surcharge to all residents' monthly charges. This freed up significant floor space in each room and improved resident morale. This approach to improving resident life_____. (p. 492)
1. Is appropriate
2. Violates Medicaid and Medicaid rules
3. Meets Medicare rules but not those of Medicaid
4. Meets Medicaid, but not Medicare rules

**66.** The resident reports the facility to the State for releasing his medical records to the local hospital. Despite his refusal to release these records when he was transferred to the local hospital. The State is like to _____. (p. 514)
1. Issue a fine
2. Inform the resident he has no right to refuse to release his records upon transfer
3. Issue a citation
4. Assure the resident it will not happen again

**67.** The resident has complained numerous times about the disruptive behavior of a nearby resident. The facility assures the resident there is nothing can be done. This is_____. (p. 493)
1. Probably an accurate statement by the facility
2. An inadequate facility response
3. A routine occurrence
4. Not addressed by Federal rules

**68.** A resident demands to see both the most recent survey results and the plan of correction. The facility shows the survey results but tells the resident that the plan of correction is confidential and not available. The facility is _____. (p. 493)
1. Within its rights
2. Violating resident rights
3. Acting prudently
4. Protecting sensitive information

## Work

**69.** The resident, upon his request, requested work delivering newspapers throughout the facility. This is an approved part of the resident's care plan. The resident receives $5.00 an hour for his work. The facility is _____. (pp. 493–494)
1. Meeting work requirements
2. Not meeting work requirements
3. Improperly documenting the resident's work
4. Appropriately humoring the resident

## Mail Rights

**70.** The resident demands computer and internet access, but the facility fails to provide this. The facility _____. (p. 494)
1. Is within its rights
2. Is failing to meet requirements
3. Is behind the times
4. Is worried about resident privacy

## Access

**71.** A representative of the Secretary knocks on the locked front door at 5:30 a.m. and wants immediate admission. The charge nurse tells the representative to wait until the facility opens at 6:00 a.m.. This is _____. (p. 494)
1. Within the facility's discretion
2. Good judgment
3. A safety and risk management behavior
4. A violation

## Furniture

72. The administrator refuses to permit a large piece of furniture to be placed in the resident's room arguing that it overly obstructs movement. The administrator is _____. (p. 494)
    1. Within his rights
    2. Ignoring resident rights
    3. Making his own rules without regard to the resident
    4. Making a mistake

## Married Couples Sharing a Room

73. Consenting married residents have a right to share a room _____. (p. 495)
    1. Regardless of their health conditions
    2. If facility policy permits
    3. When a room is conveniently available
    4. When approved by the resident council

## Self-Administration of Drugs

74. An individual resident can self-administer his drugs if _____. (p. 495)
    1. The pharmacy approves
    2. The attending physician approves
    3. The interdisciplinary team has determined this is safe
    4. The resident accepts responsibility for storing the drugs safely

## Resident Transfers

75. The facility may transfer a resident _____. (p. 489)
    1. When beds are scarce
    2. When the resident is a month late in payment of charges
    3. If the facility will close within one year
    4. If the resident is persistently disruptive to other patients comforts

76. The facility seeking to transfer a resident must _____. (p. 489)
    1. Record the reasons in the resident's clinical record
    2. Give 90 days' notice
    3. Have a good reason
    4. Need the bed for other residents who seek to return from the hospital

77. When a facility notifies a resident of a transfer on February 1, to be accomplished March 1 the facility has _____. (see Federal Requirements App. P and PP) (p. 489)
    1. Met Final Rules requirements
    2. Failed to meet Final Rules requirements
    3. Taken appropriate action when unable to meet needs
    4. Acted in good faith

78. When the nurse gives complete verbal notice of the duration of the bed-hold policy under the State plan to a resident and his family before transfer to a hospital, the facility can be said to have _____. (see Federal Requirements App. P and PP) (p. 489)
    1. Met Final Rules requirements
    2. Failed to meet Final Rules requirements
    3. Exceeded Final Rules requirements
    4. Conformed acceptably to Final Rules requirements

## Family Meetings

79. Regarding group or family meetings, after providing space and privacy to resident families and any persons they invite in, the facility obligations are _____. (see Federal Requirements App. P and PP) (p. 493)
    1. Met
    2. Partially met
    3. Exceeded
    4. Optional as to further assistance

## Private Pay

80. The facility is by policy a 100% private pay residents facility. The facility informs prospective residents both in writing and orally in a language they can understand. This_____. (p. 492)
    1. Meets the facility's obligations
    2. Is permitted under special circumstances in some Medicare certified facilities
    3. Is not permitted
    4. Is a safe business practice

## Payments

81. The facility requires only private paying patients to designate a third party who will pay the bills. Medicare and Medicaid patients are billed only from their own funds. This_____. (p. 497)
    1. Is a correct interpretation the rules
    2. Is a necessary business practice
    3. Assures a good collection rate
    4. Violates Medicare Medicaid standards

## Freedom from Restraints

82. The new administrator announces that after two weeks no restraints will be allowed, even those required to meet the residents' medical symptoms. This is _____. (p. 527)
    1. Permitted
    2. Not permitted
    3. A violation of Federal rules
    4. A mis-interpretation of the rules' intent

## Abuse

83. To lessen the risk incidents of resident abusive treatment of other residents, the facility permits Mr. Jones to remain in his room throughout the day. This is _____. (p. 490)
    1. Good risk management
    2. Within the intent of the Federal rules
    3. Abusive treatment
    4. A good way to reduce incidents of residents abusing other residents

## Restraints

84. The administrator who learns that the director of nurses obtained physicians' orders for physical restraints on three "too time-consuming 'wanderer' " residents should _____. (see Federal Requirements App. P and PP) (p. 527)
    1. Compliment the DON on solving a staffing problem
    2. Seek the same for additional residents
    3. Ask the physicians to remove the restraint orders
    4. Continue about her normal daily duties

85. An alleged violation of neglect of a resident has been lodged. The administrator has reported this to the state, conducted an investigation the next day, and concluded no violation occurred. The administrator should _____. (see Federal Requirements App. P and PP) (p. 527)
    1. Report results to state officials within 5 days of the alleged violation
    2. Document the investigation results and file it for state review at annual inspection time
    3. Reprimand the employee involved
    4. Consider the matter successfully settled

## 6.1.8 QUALITY ASSESSMENT AND ASSURANCE

86. The facility sets up mechanisms to listen to the views and record grievances and recommendations of residents and families concerning proposed policy. The facility has _____. (p. 499)
    1. Met expectations under the Federal regulation
    2. Exceeded what it is required to do
    3. Failed to meet regulations
    4. Set up a good feedback mechanism

87. A uniform data set describing the resident's capability to perform daily life functions and functional impairments is known as _____. (see Federal Requirements App. P and PP) (p. 499)
    1. The uniform (minimum) (comprehensive) data set
    2. Comprehensive care plan
    3. Resident needs assessment
    4. Resident data assessment card

**88.** Resident assessments must be conducted within _____ days after admission, after a significant mental or physical change, at least every _____ months. (see Federal Requirements App. P and PP) (p. 499)
  *1.* 6      8
  *2.* 4      6
  *3.* 14     12
  *4.* 4      24

**89.** The resident assessment must be conducted or at least coordinated by and signed by _____. (see Federal Requirements App. P and PP) (p. 499)
  *1.* The resident's physician
  *2.* The medical director or resident's physician
  *3.* A registered nurse
  *4.* The director of nursing

**90.** A resident enters a facility continent. Due to new clinical conditions, catherization becomes necessary. The facility's entire response is to provide services "to prevent urinary tract infections" and treat them if occurring. The facility has _____. (see Federal Requirements App. P and PP) (p. 499)
  *1.* Met Final Rules standards
  *2.* Failed to meet Final Rules standards
  *3.* Exceeded what is required under Final Rules
  *4.* Performed good quality care

**91.** A resident's clinical condition demonstrates that a nasogastric tube is unavoidable. The facility documents this and begins a permanent program designed to prevent aspiration pneumonia, diarrhea, vomiting, dehydration, metabolic abnormalities, and nasal-pharyngeal ulcers. A Medicare inspector would consider the facility to have _____. (see Federal Requirements App. P and PP) (p. 499)
  *1.* Met Final Rules requirements
  *2.* Exceeded Final Rules requirements
  *3.* Given excellent care
  *4.* Failed to implement the intent and spirit of Final Rules

## Roommate and Room Changes

**92.** To accommodate a resident returning from the hospital, the facility informs Mrs. Brown that in half an hour the staff will be moving in a new roommate. The facility _____. (p. 500)
  *1.* Is making the right decision
  *2.* Has the right to make such needed changes
  *3.* Is meeting its obligations to residents
  *4.* Is failing to meet its obligations to residents

## Quality Assessment and Assurance

93. The facility appoints the director of nursing, the medical director's Physician Assistant, and four additional staff members to serve on the Quality Assessment and Assurance Committee. This _____. (p. 500)
    1. Meets requirements
    2. Exceeds requirements
    3. Is optional for the facility under the new guidelines
    4. Fails to satisfy the Federal guidelines

94. The Quality Assessment and Assurance Committee chair informs the administrator that the committee meets every four months and has developed and implemented appropriate plans of action. The administrator should _____. (p. 500)
    1. Be pleased
    2. Review the written reports of this committee
    3. Be concerned
    4. Thank the chair

95. During a Medicare survey, the director of nursing refuses to disclose the records of the Quality Assessment and Assurance Committee to enable the surveyor to review the actions taken. The director of nursing is _____. (p. 500)
    1. Within her rights
    2. Acting foolishly
    3. Likely to cause an unnecessary deficiency to be given
    4. Using poor judgment

## 6.1.9 DIETARY

96. The facility identifies low potassium as a nutritional problem, provides a therapeutic diet to correct the potassium deficiency. The resident refuses the therapeutic diet and insists she wishes to eat a regular diet just like the other residents around her. The facility should _____. (p. 500)
    1. Serve the therapeutic diet
    2. Serve an enriched diet
    3. Serve a regular diet
    4. Have the resident's attending physician explain why the therapeutic diet is necessary

97. In January Mrs. Green weighed 112 pounds. In June she weighed 98 pounds. This is _____. (p. 500)
    1. Within normal weight expectations
    2. A significant weight loss
    3. A predictable weight loss
    4. A severe weight loss

## Substitutes

**98.** Mrs. Gray refused to eat the meat served for lunch. The facility offered Mrs. Brown a second salad. This is _____. (p. 501)
   *1.* Within the rules
   *2.* Appropriate
   *3.* Inappropriate
   *4.* Using good judgment since Mrs. Gray is known to especially like salads

**99.** The registered dietitian prescribes a therapeutic diet for Mrs. Blue because the dietitian noticed some weight loss in the past two months. As lunch was about to be served anyway, the kitchen staff was able to implement the new diet within 10 minutes of the nutritionist's recommendation. The administrator should _____. (p. 501)
   *1.* Feel his staff is really agile
   *2.* Meet with the dietitian
   *3.* Use this as an example of quick work at the next staff meeting
   *4.* Turn his attention to more pressing matters

**100.** During the periodic mid-afternoon visit, the consultant dietitian writes out therapeutic diets for the four new residents and hands them individually as soon as she writes them to the director of food services for preparing food for those residents that evening. Upon being informed of this that afternoon, the administrator should _____. (see Federal Requirements App. P and PP) (p. 501)
   *1.* Thank the dietitian for such fast turnaround
   *2.* Check the diets prescribed by the dietitian against the recommended nutritional needs in the Final Rules requirements
   *3.* Tell the director of food services to serve regular diets to those four new residents that night
   *4.* Permit the director of food service 2 days to implement the therapeutic diets

**101.** Snacks at bedtime _____. (see Federal Requirements App. P and PP) (p. 501)
   *1.* May be offered to competent residents
   *2.* Must be offered to all residents
   *3.* Must be nutritional if offered
   *4.* Must meet Final Rules specified nutritional values

## 6.1.10 ENVIRONMENTAL MANAGEMENT

## Preventive Maintenance

**102.** The air conditioning roof unit fan shaft has run dry and required quick oiling for several months. The facility is ____. (p. 503)
   *1.* Due for a new roof unit
   *2.* Being economical
   *3.* Practicing just in time repair
   *4.* Failing to do preventive maintenance

**103.** A facility initially certified under Final Rules, which at the request of the resident council, maintains a winter temperature of 83 degrees despite protests from staff that this is too hot for the staff is _____. (see Federal Requirements App. P and PP) (p. 503)
1. Complying with Final Rules directives
2. Not in noncompliance with Final Rules
3. Correctly responding to resident directives
4. Voluntarily exceeding the need to acceptably meet resident needs

**104.** The resident has mentioned to the administrator several times that he is tired of waiting for a room with a window to the outside. The facility is _____. (p. 503)
1. Failing to meet physical building requirements
2. Justified if no other rooms are available
3. Not doing enough to meet expectations of residents
4. Needing better policies on meeting resident room preferences

**105.** Each resident room must have _____.(see Federal Requirements App. P and PP) (p. 503)
1. A full bath
2. 125 square feet per resident
3. Its own fire extinguishment system
4. At least one window to the outside

**106.** The call systems representative's recommendations for installing a call system to the bathing facilities in addition to the present resident room and toilets call systems were turned down by the administrator as too expensive. This _____. (p. 503)
1. Is the administrator's prerogative
2. Is reasonable in light of reimbursement levels
3. Meets enough requirements without the additional call system
4. Is not meeting standards

## 6.1.11 INFECTION CONTROL

**107.** The facility has an infection control program that has effectively investigated and controlled every infectious outbreak. When the state visits and evaluates this program the state will likely _____. (p. 504)
1. Be pleased
2. See this an example to be recommended
3. Issue a deficiency
4. Ask about how this has been so successfully accomplished

**108.** Such details as size of committee, scope of work, and reporting requirements for the infection control function are _____. (see Federal Requirements App. P and PP) (p. 504)
1. Carefully described in Final Rules
2. Left to the facility
3. Left to the individual states to specify
4. Recommended but not required under Final Rules

109. Maintaining a record of incidents and corrective actions related to infections is assigned under Final Rules to _____. (see Federal Requirements App. P and PP) (p. 504)
   1. The nursing department
   2. The medical director
   3. The infection control program
   4. A mandated quality control coordinator

110. The general approach of the Federal Requirements is to state federal requirements, for example, infection control, and budgets required, _____. (see Federal Requirements App. P and PP) (p. 504)
   1. In general (less specific or detailed) terms
   2. In great detail
   3. To achieve closer control
   4. To insure identical policies facility to facility

## 6.1.12 PHYSICIAN SERVICES

111. The nurse was miffed that she could not get a medical decision until the attending physician was to return from a medical convention and mentions this to the administrator. The administrator should _____. (p. 505)
   1. Meet immediately with the director of nursing
   2. Assure the resident a decision is being made as soon as practicable
   3. Reprimand the nurse
   4. Suggest the nurse improve her self-control

112. A physician visit occurring 14 days after the date the visit was required is _____. (see Federal Requirements App. P and PP) (p. 505)
   1. Not considered timely
   2. Considered timely
   3. Permitted occasionally
   4. Routinely permitted

113. If a facility policy prohibits use of physician assistants, but three physicians routinely use physician assistants for most visits, the Medicare inspector will _____. (see Federal Requirements App. P and PP) (p. 506)
   1. Approve the procedure as a Medicare authorized care procedure
   2. Cite the facility
   3. Ascertain the acceptability to the residents concerned of use of physician assistants
   4. Encourage such cost savings to Medicare

114. Ultimate responsibility for obtaining and reporting laboratory, radiology, and other diagnostic services is assigned to the _____. (see Federal Requirements App. P and PP) (p. 506)
   1. Medical director
   2. Nursing facility
   3. Attending physician issuing the orders
   4. Attending physician's office staff

115. The charge nurse notices that lab work recommended for a particular medication has not been ordered and places the order. The administrator should _____. (see Federal Requirements App. P and PP) (p. 506)
    1. Sign off on the order
    2. Praise the nurse
    3. Document the order
    4. Be upset

116. A facility need not first consult with the resident or the resident's physician when there is _____.(see Federal Requirements App. P and PP) (p. 506)
    1. An accident involving injury
    2. A decision to transfer
    3. A change in roommate
    4. A medical emergency

117. The medical director declined to take responsibility for monitoring and ensuring implementation of resident care policies feeling this was too time consuming. The administrator would be well advised to _____. (p. 506)
    1. Agree with the medical director
    2. Enter a complaint to the state about the medical director
    3. Find a new medical director
    4. Assign that task to the director of nursing

118. Upon learning that, to save expenses, the director of nurses has determined that drug records are in order and that all controlled drugs are accounted for, the administrator should _____. (see Federal Requirements App. P and PP) (p. 506)
    1. Be pleased and compliment the DON
    2. Thank the DON for the information and continue about his/her business
    3. Call the consulting pharmacist
    4. Plan an inservice for other nurses

119. Permitting a resident, whose physician permits drugs judged unnecessary but demanded by the resident, to continue to take unnecessary drugs _____. (see Federal Requirements App. P and PP) (p. 506)
    1. Is encouraged
    2. Is generally acceptable
    3. Is not permitted
    4. Is permitted if the resident self-administers drugs

120. New facilities certified under Final Rules must meet the applicable provisions of the _____. (see Federal Requirements App. P and PP) (p. 506)
    1. National Fire Protection Association
    2. Occupational Safety and Health Act as amended
    3. *Life Safety Code* of 2000
    4. *Life Safety Code* of 1990

## Plan D

**121.** Plan D, implemented in 2008, was intended to _____. (see Federal Requirements App. P and PP) (p. 523)
1. Provide stricter oversight of care
2. Provide relief from medication expenses
3. Cover outlier costs
4. Decrease federal involvement

## Nurses Aide Training

**122.** An individual who can prove he or she recently successfully completed a training and competency evaluation program, but who is not actually registered in the required registry _____ as a nurses aide. (see Federal Requirements App. P and PP) (p. 484)
1. Can be hired
2. Must not be hired
3. Is temporarily eligible for hiring
4. Is likely overqualified

**123.** Responsibility for determining whether the nurses aide training and competency evaluation requirements are met in a facility falls to the _____. (see Federal Requirements App. P and PP) (p. 484)
1. Medicare inspectors
2. Medicaid inspectors
3. State Nursing Board
4. State survey agency

**124.** The owner of a facility providing nearly the best nurses aide training and competency evaluation program in the state declines to permit an unannounced visit by the State. The State will _____. (see Federal Requirements App. P and PP) (p. 484)
1. Return at a more acceptable time
2. Withdraw approval of the training program
3. Make an announced visit within 5 working days
4. Make an announced visit within 10 working days

**125.** The required curriculum for a nurses aide training program does not have to include _____. (see Federal Requirements App. P and PP) (p. 484)
1. Basic nursing skills
2. Personal care skills
3. Care of cognitively impaired residents
4. Diet management

**126.** Candidates for nurses aide competency evaluation are normally examined by _____. (see Federal Requirements App. P and PP) (p. 484)
1. A Medicare participating skilled nursing facility
2. A Medicaid nursing facility
3. The individual's own facility
4. A State-approved entity

**127.** Under federal guidelines a candidate for nurses aide registration has _____ chances to take the evaluation. (see Federal Requirements App. P and PP) (p. 484)
   *1.* Two
   *2.* No more than three
   *3.* Four
   *4.* At least three

**128.** A finding by the State survey agency of abuse or neglect by a nurses aide remains recorded in the nurse aide registry _____. (see Federal Requirements App. P and PP) (p. 484)
   *1.* For 2 years
   *2.* For 4 years
   *3.* Forever
   *4.* During the recommended probation period

**129.** Ensuring that nurse aides are able to demonstrate competency in skills and techniques necessary to care for residents' needs is the responsibility of _____. (see Federal Requirements App. P and PP) (p. 484)
   *1.* The State
   *2.* Medicaid program officials
   *3.* Medicare officials
   *4.* The facility

## 6.1.13 DENTAL SERVICES

**130.** Under Final Rules, routine and emergency dental services are _____. (see Federal Requirements App. P and PP) (p. 507)
   *1.* Optional
   *2.* Mandated
   *3.* Upon request of the resident
   *4.* Upon order of the resident's physician

## 6.1.14 NURSING POLICIES

**131.** The director of nursing mentions to the administrator that although Ms. Brown had no significant change in her physical or mental condition upon readmission, a full comprehensive assessment was completed within 5 days of her return. The administrator might feel _____. (p. 507)
   *1.* Facility resources might not be
      utilized efficiently
   *2.* Satisfied that effectiveness had been achieved
   *3.* Pleased that the assessment was within the 14 day window
   *4.* Alarmed

**132.** To stretch resources, the care planning team decides to conduct comprehensive assessments on the healthiest patients every 15 months. The administrator should feel_____. (p. 507)
1. That the staff is making a reasonable choice
2. The staff is being proactive
3. A deficiency is in his future
4. The care team has saved the facility some expenditures

## Standards of Quality

**133.** Standards of quality for care given in the nursing facility _____. (p. 508)
1. May be found in several venues
2. Come only from CMS
3. Are those set out in the Federal Requirements
4. Can be developed by the facility or its parent body

### 6.1.15 QUALITY OF CARE USING THE RAI

**134.** The nurse on duty has informed Ms. Brown that Ms. Brown must make arrangements for transportation to her audiologist. This is_____. (p. 511)
1. Correct
2. Not permitted facility policy
3. Prudent shepherding of facility staff time
4. A realistic response

**135.** Psychosocial adjustment difficulties _____. (p, 510)
1. Are inevitable
2. Are not common in today's environment
3. Are the responsibility of the resident
4. Must be treated by the facility

**136.** For several months in succession it is noted in the resident's records that the resident is becoming more withdrawn. The facility _____. (p. 510)
1. Has met its record keeping requirements
2. Should show more staff interest in this resident
3. Must develop a plan of care to address this
4. Should provide more opportunities for interaction among the residents

**137.** For nasogastrically fed patients, the facility program is to provide treatment and services to prevent aspiration, pneumonia, diarrhea, vomiting, dehydration, and metabolic abnormalities. This _____. (pp. 510–511)
1. Is satisfactory
2. Is more than required
3. Meets minimum standards
4. Is insufficient

**138.** Ms. Green has been shouting incoherently at nearby residents. Her physician prescribes an antipsychotic drug to calm her down. This _____. (p. 512)
1. Is reasonable
2. Is necessary for the comfort of the other residents
3. Is unacceptable
4. Follows usual medical practice decisions

## 6.1.16 PHARMACY

**139.** The facility must provide a separately locked, permanently affixed compart-
ment for storage of controlled drugs listed in Schedule _____ of the Drug Act.
(p. 513)
1. I
2. II
3. III
4. V

**140.** Controlled drugs listed in Schedule I of the Comprehensive Drug Abuse Act of
1970 are _____. (see Federal Requirements App. P and PP) (p. 512)
1. To be kept locked
2. To be kept locked and under proper temperature controls
3. Not permitted in the facility
4. Used only on the order of a licensed physician

### 6.1.17 Medical Records

**141.** The administrator's policy is to discard all clinical records after ten years. This policy is _____. (p. 514)
1. In accordance with requirements
2. Practical: meets all possible state and federal requirements
3. Flawed
4. Causing unduly long retention of records

# 6.2
# Developing a Care Plan

### Resident Assessment Instrument

**142.** The Resident Assessment Instrument is a set of screening, clinical, and functional
status elements that form the basis for _____. (p. 515)
1. A comprehensive assessment of each resident
2. A thorough plan of care
3. Improving reimbursement
4. Capacity for a look-back in care needs

**143.** Specific resident responses for one or a combination of MDS elements are _____. (p. 515)
1. The minimum elements
2. The RAI
3. The Care Area Triggers
4. The care plan

**144.** The MDS care planning process can be visualized as: assessment, decision making, and _____. (p. 515)
1. Follow-up
2. Visualization of resident needs
3. Documentation of resident preferences
4. Care plan

# 6.3
# The Survey

**145.** In planning an annual survey the surveyor begins with reviewing current government data records on the facility, current complaints, Ombudsman information, and _____. (p. 519)
1. The facility care plans
2. The comprehensive assessments
3. Current MDS data
4. All OSCAR data

**146.** The surveyors expect information on contact persons for complaints or abuse, a list of ventilator dependent residents, a list of residents on hospice, a list of dialysis patients within _____ hours of entering a facility for survey. (p. 519)
1. One day
2. One hour
3. Four hours
4. 24 hours

**147.** The administrator can expect surveyors to generate _____ lists of residents to be interviewed. (p. 519)
1. Two
2. Eight
3. Three or more
4. Six

148. As a matter of policy, at the Exit Conference _____ are/is invited to attend. (p. 520)
    1. All resident council members
    2. The resident council president
    3. Any interested residents
    4. Only invited residents

149. If a facility plan of correction is found unacceptable _____. (p. 520)
    1. The facility is fined
    2. A fast-track process will begin
    3. The facility can appeal
    4. A new plan of correction must be submitted

150. Normally, a plan of correction _____. (p. 520)
    1. Is accepted by the state
    2. Meets requirements
    3. Triggers a revisit
    4. Is appealed

151. Hoping to delay an enforcement action, the administrator asks for an Informal Dispute Resolution. The administrator _____. (p. 521)
    1. Does not understand the process
    2. Has made a prudent move
    3. Is taking advisable defensive action
    4. Will likely win at least half the time

# 6.4
# The Surveyors' Findings

152. A finding by surveyors that in both wings of the facility the water to resident rooms and baths is 8 degrees above the upper limit, but that no one had yet been burned, would result in a deficiency characterized as _____. (p. 521)
    1. Broad and high
    2. Widespread
    3. Widespread, no actual harm with minimum potential for actual harm
    4. Widespread, no actual harm with potential for more than minimal harm

# 6.5
# Reimbursement for Care Given

## PPS

**153.** The CMS goal is to reimburse based on how much _____ is required to care for each patient each month. (p. 522)
1. Money
2. Staff in place
3. Effort
4. Staff time

**154.** There are _____ levels and types of care for reimbursing nursing facility care given. (p. 522)
1. Increasing diverse
2. Sixty-six
3. Fifteen
4. Five broad categories of

## MDS

**155.** The MDS contains items that reflect the _____ of the resident. (p. 523)
1. Activity level
2. Ability to pay
3. General circumstances
4. Acuity level

**156.** The Medicare-required assessments provide information about the clinical condition of beneficiaries. These assessments _____. (p. 523)
1. Can be scheduled in advance
2. Can be unscheduled
3. Can be scheduled or unscheduled
4. Can be known in advance

**157.** Readmission/return assessment, start of therapy, and end of therapy are _____. (p. 523)
1. Excluded from standardized assessment dates
2. Standardized assessment dates
3. The 5-, 14-, 30-, 60-, 90- day assessments
4. More highly reimbursed

## RUG Classification

**158.** The RUG-IV classification system has _____ major categories. (p. 523)
1. Four
2. Eight
3. Twelve
4. A varying number of

**159.** The scheduled PPS assessments (performed around Day 5, 14, 30, 60, and 90) establish _____ for associated standard payment periods. (p. 523)
   *1.* A little used basis
   *2.* A free moving basis
   *3.* Per diem payment rates
   *4.* Monthly rates

## ADLs

**160.** The ADL score is based upon the ADLs:_____. (p. 523)
   *1.* Bed mobility, activities, toilet use, and ambulating
   *2.* Transferring, eating, and activities
   *3.* Walking, bed mobility, and eating
   *4.* Bed mobility, transfer, toilet use, and eating

## Reimbursement

**161.** A cancer patient receiving intensive therapies may _____. (p. 523)
   *1.* Be a good source of extra revenue
   *2.* Be an ideal admission
   *3.* Cost the facility more than it will be reimbursed
   *4.* Increase facility cash flow positively

**162.** The current long-term health care delivery system is one in which each player seeks to minimize its own costs at the possible expense of _____. (p. 524)
   *1.* The taxpayers
   *2.* Private paying patients
   *3.* The revenue base
   *4.* Other players in the system

**163.** How much a facility can charge for care given can be characterized as _____. (p. 524)
   *1.* A given
   *2.* Easy to chart
   *3.* A simple computer algorithm
   *4.* A moving target

**164.** Establishing transfer and discharge policies according to source of payment _____ under Final Rules. (see Federal Requirements App. P and PP) (p. 497)
   *1.* Is permitted
   *2.* Is discouraged
   *3.* Is forbidden
   *4.* Must be fully documented

**1.** (2) During 1998 and 1999, the price paid per bed in nursing home purchases tended to be too high to sustain over the following years when reimbursements were squeezed by Medicare and Medicaid.

**2.** (2) It is nearly always desirable to be efficient as well as effective.

**3.** (2) The administrator fails to anticipate that the occupancy rate of the facility is likely to fall and that, in any case, with the new competition, a new approach to admissions will most likely be necessary. The administrator is failing to react appropriately to changes in the environment that will likely impact the facility.

**4.** (3) From the founding of the large scale nursing home industry in the 1960s until the year 2000 very few bankruptcies were experienced.

**5.** (2) Medicare (and Medicaid) forced facilities to give more services for a single re-imbursement rate than had been the case previously.

**6.** (2) Medicare, to cut its own costs, has required facilities to give more services under the Medicare reimbursement given.

**7.** (4) The director of nursing fails to understand that using expensive RN hours, when less expensive LPN and CNA hours, are the industry standard will be unsustainably expensive for the facility.

**8.** (4) Case mix in the typical rural facility is hard to manipulate, but in the teaching hospital setting the facility normally must maximize the number of Medicare rehabilitation patients in order to remain competitive and solvent.

**9.** (4) The DON normally reports directly to the administrator. The assistant administrator wants too much power or does not understand how normal nursing facilities function.

**10.** (2) Under bankruptcy plans the court assures that all current bills are paid. The medical supplies provider does not understand the bankruptcy laws.

**11.** (3) MBWA, to be effective, must be done daily; weekly is too infrequent.

**12.** (4) It is normally better to go through the chain of command and let the employees' immediate supervisor request the corrections.

**13.** (1) A number of market forces have held down any significant building of new facilities in recent years. This may change.

**14.** (4) The successful nursing home administrator will need to employ several administrative styles to get the facility's work successfully accomplished.

**15.** (1) This candidate understands the need for flexibility in leadership styles and believes he has successfully used several styles.

**16.** (2) Charismatic leadership is given to leaders by followers. A leader cannot just declare herself charismatic.

**17.** (1) Yes, acute care reimbursement rates are higher than average, but so are the costs!

**18.** (4) It is impossible to prevent informal communications among nurses and the nurse supervisor seems to not have enough communication savvy to understand this.

**19.** (2) The department head understands that employees often engage in selective hearing; that is, hearing good news and screening out anything unpleasant.

**20.** (4) The administrator must get information from all levels of management in order to know what is actually going on. It is dangerous to rely solely on one person.

**21.** (4) Nursing shortages come and go, but mostly there is a seemingly chronic shortage of good nurse candidates.

**22.** (1) It is impossible and undesirable to try to write enough rules to make every facility function successfully.

**23.** (1) It is normal for the various department such as nursing, housekeeping, and dietary to seek to "turn over" as much work to other departments as they can.

**24.** (1) The administrator may have all reports made available to him, but requiring that he see all reports before signed would likely be dysfunctional for getting the facility's work done in a timely manner.

**25.** (3) Correctly filled out incident reports is a must for the facility, and this situation is not likely to "correct itself" without the administrator's active intervention.

**26.** (1) Corporate wants that facility to have as nearly a deficiency free inspection as possible and is willing to pay a little more for that year's performance to achieve this.

**27.** (1) In recent years, federal and state governments have been seeking to reduce the proportion of funds that go to institutional care.

**28.** (3) This was a part of the effort a few years ago to get nursing facilities reimbursed for the actual costs incurred in giving care.

**29.** (2) Expect that efforts to shift cost from Medicare and Medicaid onto facilities will continue.

**30.** (1) The residents may in fact get better care, but if it is not documented, the survey team has no real way to give credit for the care given. Give excellent care, but also document, document, document.

**31.** (3) The social worker has to do both if assigned both. The social worker needs to renegotiate her job description with the administrator.

# ANSWER KEY

## 1. NAB DOMAIN: MANAGEMENT, GOVERNANCE, LEADERSHIP

**LEARNING HOW TO MANAGE THE
HEALTH CARE ORGANIZATION**

| | | | | | | | | |
|---|---|---|---|---|---|---|---|---|
| 1. *2* | 29. *2* | 57. *3* | 85. *3* | 113. *4* | 141. *4* | 169. *1* | 197. *4* | 225. *3* |
| 2. *2* | 30. *1* | 58. *3* | 86. *1* | 114. *4* | 142. *3* | 170. *1* | 198. *4* | 226. *2* |
| 3. *2* | 31. *3* | 59. *1* | 87. *2* | 115. *4* | 143. *3* | 171. *4* | 199. *2* | 227. *3* |
| 4. *3* | 32. *3* | 60. *1* | 88. *4* | 116. *3* | 144. *3* | 172. *3* | 200. *2* | 228. *3* |
| 5. *2* | 33. *3* | 61. *2* | 89. *1* | 117. *3* | 145. *4* | 173. *3* | 201. *2* | 229. *2* |
| 6. *2* | 34. *3* | 62. *2* | 90. *2* | 118. *1* | 146. *4* | 174. *4* | 202. *2* | 230. *1* |
| 7. *4* | 35. *2* | 63. *3* | 91. *3* | 119. *3* | 147. *4* | 175. *2* | 203. *3* | 231. *3* |
| 8. *4* | 36. *3* | 64. *4* | 92. *1* | 120. *2* | 148. *4* | 176. *3* | 204. *3* | 232. *1* |
| 9. *4* | 37. *2* | 65. *1* | 93. *3* | 121. *3* | 149. *1* | 177. *4* | 205. *1* | 233. *3* |
| 10. *2* | 38. *3* | 66. *4* | 94. *4* | 122. *3* | 150. *1* | 178. *2* | 206. *3* | 234. *2* |
| 11. *3* | 39. *2* | 67. *1* | 95. *3* | 123. *4* | 151. *1* | 179. *4* | 207. *2* | 235. *1* |
| 12. *4* | 40. *4* | 68. *3* | 96. *3* | 124. *1* | 152. *1* | 180. *4* | 208. *3* | 236. *4* |
| 13. *1* | 41. *3* | 69. *2* | 97. *4* | 125. *3* | 153. *3* | 181. *4* | 209. *3* | 237. *3* |
| 14. *4* | 42. *1* | 70. *2* | 98. *4* | 126. *1* | 154. *4* | 182. *3* | 210. *3* | 238. *4* |
| 15. *1* | 43. *2* | 71. *3* | 99. *4* | 127. *3* | 155. *3* | 183. *3* | 211. *3* | 239. *3* |
| 16. *2* | 44. *1* | 72. *2* | 100. *2* | 128. *1* | 156. *2* | 184. *3* | 212. *1* | 240. *2* |
| 17. *1* | 45. *2* | 73. *1* | 101. *1* | 129. *4* | 157. *4* | 185. *4* | 213. *3* | 241. *3* |
| 18. *4* | 46. *2* | 74. *3* | 102. *2* | 130. *1* | 158. *2* | 186. *4* | 214. *3* | 242. *4* |
| 19. *2* | 47. *1* | 75. *3* | 103. *3* | 131. *2* | 159. *2* | 187. *1* | 215. *2* | 243. *2* |
| 20. *4* | 48. *1* | 76. *1* | 104. *4* | 132. *2* | 160. *1* | 188. *3* | 216. *1* | 244. *4* |
| 21. *4* | 49. *3* | 77. *3* | 105. *1* | 133. *3* | 161. *1* | 189. *3* | 217. *4* | 245. *1* |
| 22. *1* | 50. *3* | 78. *3* | 106. *1* | 134. *1* | 162. *4* | 190. *4* | 218. *3* | 246. *2* |
| 23. *1* | 51. *2* | 79. *4* | 107. *1* | 135. *1* | 163. *1* | 191. *3* | 219. *2* | 247. *1* |
| 24. *1* | 52. *4* | 80. *4* | 108. *3* | 136. *2* | 164. *2* | 192. *4* | 220. *4* | 248. *4* |
| 25. *3* | 53. *1* | 81. *3* | 109. *3* | 137. *3* | 165. *3* | 193. *1* | 221. *1* | 249. *3* |
| 26. *1* | 54. *4* | 82. *2* | 110. *3* | 138. *1* | 166. *2* | 194. *2* | 222. *3* | 250. *3* |
| 27. *1* | 55. *3* | 83. *4* | 111. *3* | 139. *2* | 167. *3* | 195. *4* | 223. *3* | |
| 28. *3* | 56. *1* | 84. *3* | 112. *2* | 140. *3* | 168. *2* | 196. *3* | 224. *3* | |

## 2. NAB DOMAIN: HUMAN RESOURCES

### UNDERSTANDING THE DEPARTMENTS AND MANAGING HUMAN RESOURCES

| | | | | | | | | |
|---|---|---|---|---|---|---|---|---|
| 1. *1* | 16. *1* | 31. *3* | 46. *3* | 61. *1* | 76. *2* | 91. *4* | 106. *4* | 121. *1* |
| 2. *2* | 17. *4* | 32. *3* | 47. *3* | 62. *2* | 77. *1* | 92. *4* | 107. *4* | 122. *3* |
| 3. *1* | 18. *4* | 33. *1* | 48. *2* | 62. *1* | 78. *3* | 93. *3* | 108. *4* | 123. *4* |
| 4. *4* | 19. *1* | 34. *4* | 49. *2* | 64. *1* | 79. *3* | 94. *4* | 109. *3* | 124. *4* |
| 5. *3* | 20. *1* | 35. *3* | 50. *4* | 65. *1* | 80. *4* | 95. *2* | 110. *4* | 125. *2* |
| 6. *3* | 21. *2* | 36. *2* | 51. *1* | 66. *4* | 81. *4* | 96. *2* | 111. *3* | 126. *3* |
| 7. *4* | 22. *3* | 37. *3* | 52. *3* | 67. *2* | 82. *4* | 97. *1* | 112. *3* | 127. *2* |
| 8. *4* | 23. *4* | 38. *1* | 53. *1* | 68. *1* | 83. *3* | 98. *2* | 113. *1* | 128. *4* |
| 9. *4* | 24. *3* | 39. *3* | 54. *1* | 69. *2* | 84. *4* | 99. *4* | 114. *3* | 129. *2* |
| 10. *4* | 25. *3* | 40. *4* | 55. *4* | 70. *1* | 85. *4* | 100. *4* | 115. *1* | 130. *4* |
| 11. *3* | 26. *4* | 41. *3* | 56. *4* | 71. *4* | 86. *3* | 101. *1* | 116. *3* | 131. *3* |
| 12. *1* | 27. *2* | 42. *3* | 57. *4* | 72. *2* | 87. *3* | 102. *1* | 117. *4* | 132. *4* |
| 13. *1* | 28. *1* | 43. *2* | 58. *1* | 73. *4* | 88. *4* | 103. *2* | 118. *4* | 133. *3* |
| 14. *2* | 29. *1* | 44. *3* | 59. *1* | 74. *3* | 89. *4* | 104. *2* | 119. *4* | 134. *2* |
| 15. *1* | 30. *4* | 45. *3* | 60. *1* | 75. *3* | 90. *4* | 105. *3* | 120. *1* | |

## 3. NAB DOMAIN: FINANCE AND BUSINESS

### LEARNING TO MANAGE THE ORGANIZATION'S FINANCES

| | | | | | | | | |
|---|---|---|---|---|---|---|---|---|
| 1. *2* | 13. *1* | 25. *1* | 37. *3* | 49. *3* | 61. *2* | 73. *2* | 85. *3* | 97. *1* |
| 2. *3* | 14. *3* | 26. *3* | 38. *2* | 50. *1* | 62. *2* | 74. *2* | 86. *2* | 98. *4* |
| 3. *1* | 15. *1* | 27. *2* | 39. *1* | 51. *2* | 63. *3* | 75. *3* | 87. *3* | 99. *4* |
| 4. *4* | 16. *1* | 28. *4* | 40. *2* | 52. *4* | 64. *1* | 76. *3* | 88. *3* | 100. *4* |
| 5. *1* | 17. *1* | 29. *2* | 41. *1* | 53. *1* | 65. *2* | 77. *2* | 89. *2* | |
| 6. *2* | 18. *3* | 30. *1* | 42. *2* | 54. *1* | 66. *3* | 78. *2* | 90. *3* | |
| 7. *2* | 19. *2* | 31. *4* | 43. *1* | 55. *3* | 67. *2* | 79. *1* | 91. *3* | |
| 8. *4* | 20. *4* | 32. *2* | 44. *3* | 56. *3* | 68. *1* | 80. *4* | 92. *4* | |
| 9. *3* | 21. *3* | 33. *4* | 45. *2* | 57. *1* | 69. *2* | 81. *2* | 93. *3* | |
| 10. *2* | 22. *1* | 34. *1* | 46. *1* | 58. *3* | 70. *1* | 82. *1* | 94. *3* | |
| 11. *1* | 23. *3* | 35. *3* | 47. *3* | 59. *3* | 71. *2* | 83. *3* | 95. *2* | |
| 12. *2* | 24. *4* | 36. *1* | 48. *3* | 60. *4* | 72. *1* | 84. *2* | 96. *1* | |

## LEGAL AND BUSINESS TERMINOLOGY

| | | | | | | | |
|---|---|---|---|---|---|---|---|
| 1. *4* | 5. *2* | 9. *2* | 13. *1* | 17. *2* | 21. *1* | 25. *4* | 29. *4* |
| 2. *2* | 6. *1* | 10. *1* | 14. *2* | 18. *1* | 22. *2* | 26. *4* | 30. *1* |
| 3. *1* | 7. *3* | 11. *2* | 15. *1* | 19. *3* | 23. *1* | 27. *1* | 31. *1* |
| 4. *4* | 8. *1* | 12. *2* | 16. *1* | 20. *1* | 24. *2* | 28. *3* | 32. *1* |

## 4. NAB DOMAIN: ENVIRONMENT: LEARNING THE LONG-TERM CARE CONTINUUM

## INDUSTRY OVERVIEW

| | | | |
|---|---|---|---|
| 1. *2* | 3. *4* | 5. *4* | 7. *2* |
| 2. *2* | 4. *2* | 6. *2* | 8. *2* |

## REGULATIONS

| | | | | | | | |
|---|---|---|---|---|---|---|---|
| 1. *1* | 9. *3* | 17. *2* | 25. *1* | 33. *2* | 41. *3* | 49. *2* | 57. *4* |
| 2. *4* | 10. *1* | 18. *1* | 26. *4* | 34. *3* | 42. *1* | 50. *4* | 58. *3* |
| 3. *4* | 11. *4* | 19. *2* | 27. *1* | 35. *1* | 43. *1* | 51. *4* | 59. *2* |
| 4. *3* | 12. *4* | 20. *2* | 28. *1* | 36. *1* | 44. *2* | 52. *1* | 60. *2* |
| 5. *2* | 13. *3* | 21. *4* | 29. *4* | 37. *3* | 45. *4* | 53. *1* | 61. *2* |
| 6. *4* | 14. *1* | 22. *1* | 30. *3* | 38. *2* | 46. *2* | 54. *1* | 62. *1* |
| 7. *4* | 15. *3* | 23. *1* | 31. *2* | 39. *1* | 47. *1* | 55. *3* | 63. *4* |
| 8. *3* | 16. *1* | 24. *2* | 32. *4* | 40. *4* | 48. *1* | 56. *2* | 64. *1* |

## 5. NAB DOMAIN: RESIDENT/PATIENT CARE BUILDING YOUR RESIDENT CARE SKILLS

### THE AGING PROCESS OVERVIEW, THEORIES

| | | |
|---|---|---|
| **1.** *2* | **3.** *4* | **5.** *1* |
| **2.** *2* | **4.** *1* | **6.** *1* |

### MEDICAL AND RELATED TERMS: SPECIALIZATIONS

| | | | | | | | |
|---|---|---|---|---|---|---|---|
| **1.** *3* | **3.** *4* | **5.** *3* | **7.** *3* | **9.** *1* | **11.** *3* | **13.** *2* | **15.** *2* |
| **2.** *4* | **4.** *3* | **6.** *2* | **8.** *1* | **10.** *1* | **12.** *2* | **14.** *1* | |

### THERAPEUTIC ACTIONS OF DRUGS

| | | | | | | | |
|---|---|---|---|---|---|---|---|
| **1.** *2* | **3.** *1* | **5.** *1* | **7.** *4* | **9.** *1* | **11.** *2* | **13.** *3* | **15.** *2* |
| **2.** *1* | **4.** *1* | **6.** *4* | **8.** *3* | **10.** *4* | **12.** *4* | **14.** *4* | **16.** *2* |

### ABBREVIATIONS

| | | | | | | | | |
|---|---|---|---|---|---|---|---|---|
| **1.** *1* | **5.** *4* | **9.** *1* | **13.** *2* | **17.** *1* | **21.** *3* | **25.** *2* | **29.** *3* | **33.** *4* |
| **2.** *2* | **6.** *1* | **10.** *1* | **14.** *3* | **18.** *1* | **22.** *2* | **26.** *3* | **30.** *3* | **34.** *2* |
| **3.** *2* | **7.** *3* | **11.** *1* | **15.** *2* | **19.** *3* | **23.** *1* | **27.** *1* | **31.** *1* | **35.** *3* |
| **4.** *4* | **8.** *4* | **12.** *3* | **16.** *4* | **20.** *1* | **24.** *4* | **28.** *2* | **32.** *1* | |

### PREFIXES

| | | | | | | | | |
|---|---|---|---|---|---|---|---|---|
| **1.** *1* | **7.** *2* | **13.** *1* | **19.** *4* | **25.** *1* | **31.** *2* | **37.** *3* | **43.** *3* | **49.** *2* |
| **2.** *1* | **8.** *4* | **14.** *4* | **20.** *4* | **26.** *4* | **32.** *1* | **38.** *1* | **44.** *1* | **50.** *1* |
| **3.** *4* | **9.** *2* | **15.** *4* | **21.** *1* | **27.** *2* | **33.** *2* | **39.** *4* | **45.** *1* | |
| **4.** *2* | **10.** *4* | **16.** *3* | **22.** *1* | **28.** *2* | **34.** *1* | **40.** *2* | **46.** *1* | |
| **5.** *1* | **11.** *2* | **17.** *1* | **23.** *1* | **29.** *3* | **35.** *4* | **41.** *2* | **47.** *3* | |
| **6.** *4* | **12.** *4* | **18.** *1* | **24.** *2* | **30.** *3* | **36.** *1* | **42.** *2* | **48.** *2* | |

## SUFFIXES

| | | | | | |
|---|---|---|---|---|---|
| 1. *3* | 5. *3* | 9. *2* | 13. *1* | 17. *4* | 21. *2* |
| 2. *4* | 6. *2* | 10. *1* | 14. *2* | 18. *3* | 22. *3* |
| 3. *4* | 7. *4* | 11. *1* | 15. *2* | 19. *1* | 23. *2* |
| 4. *4* | 8. *4* | 12. *4* | 16. *4* | 20. *1* | |

## DISEASES

| | | | | | | | | |
|---|---|---|---|---|---|---|---|---|
| 1. *4* | 8. *2* | 15. *4* | 22. *2* | 29. *4* | 36. *2* | 43. *1* | 50. *3* | 57. *3* |
| 2. *3* | 9. *2* | 16. *2* | 23. *4* | 30. *1* | 37. *4* | 44. *2* | 51. *1* | 58. *2* |
| 3. *1* | 10. *3* | 17. *2* | 24. *1* | 31. *1* | 38. *2* | 45. *1* | 52. *3* | 59. *2* |
| 4. *4* | 11. *3* | 18. *3* | 25. *3* | 32. *4* | 39. *2* | 46. *4* | 53. *3* | 60. *1* |
| 5. *1* | 12. *1* | 19. *2* | 26. *3* | 33. *3* | 40. *4* | 47. *1* | 54. *3* | |
| 6. *4* | 13. *1* | 20. *2* | 27. *1* | 34. *2* | 41. *4* | 48. *1* | 55. *1* | |
| 7. *2* | 14. *2* | 21. *4* | 28. *4* | 35. *1* | 42. *2* | 49. *1* | 56. *4* | |

## 6. PUTTING THE SYSTEM TOGETHER

| | | | | | | | | |
|---|---|---|---|---|---|---|---|---|
| 1. *2* | 20. *2* | 39. *4* | 58. *2* | 77. *2* | 96. *2* | 115. *4* | 134. *2* | 153. *4* |
| 2. *3* | 21. *2* | 40. *2* | 59. *2* | 78. *2* | 97. *4* | 116. *4* | 135. *4* | 154. *2* |
| 3. *2* | 22. *2* | 41. *1* | 60. *1* | 79. *2* | 98. *3* | 117. *3* | 136. *3* | 155. *4* |
| 4. *4* | 23. *1* | 42. *4* | 61. *3* | 80. *3* | 99. *2* | 118. *3* | 137. *4* | 156. *3* |
| 5. *2* | 24. *3* | 43. *3* | 62. *1* | 81. *4* | 100. *3* | 119. *3* | 138. *3* | 157. *2* |
| 6. *3* | 25. *1* | 44. *4* | 63. *3* | 82. *1* | 101. *2* | 120. *3* | 139. *2* | 158. *2* |
| 7. *2* | 26. *1* | 45. *3* | 64. *4* | 83. *3* | 102. *4* | 121. *2* | 140. *3* | 159. *3* |
| 8. *4* | 27. *3* | 46. *2* | 65. *2* | 84. *3* | 103. *2* | 122. *1* | 141. *3* | 160. *4* |
| 9. *1* | 28. *3* | 47. *1* | 66. *2* | 85. *1* | 104. *1* | 123. *4* | 142. *1* | 161. *3* |
| 10. *3* | 29. *2* | 48. *2* | 67. *2* | 86. *3* | 105. *4* | 124. *2* | 143. *3* | 162. *4* |
| 11. *1* | 30. *4* | 49. *4* | 68. *2* | 87. *1* | 106. *4* | 125. *4* | 144. *4* | 163. *4* |
| 12. *3* | 31. *4* | 50. *2* | 69. *2* | 88. *3* | 107. *3* | 126. *4* | 145. *3* | 164. *3* |
| 13. *4* | 32. *2* | 51. *4* | 70. *1* | 89. *3* | 108. *2* | 127. *4* | 146. *3* | |
| 14. *3* | 33. *2* | 52. *4* | 71. *4* | 90. *2* | 109. *3* | 128. *3* | 147. *3* | |
| 15. *3* | 34. *4* | 53. *3* | 72. *1* | 91. *4* | 110. *1* | 129. *4* | 148. *2* | |
| 16. *2* | 35. *2* | 54. *3* | 73. *1* | 92. *4* | 111. *1* | 130. *2* | 149. *4* | |
| 17. *4* | 36. *3* | 55. *2* | 74. *3* | 93. *4* | 112. *2* | 131. *1* | 150. *3* | |
| 18. *4* | 37. *4* | 56. *3* | 75. *3* | 94. *3* | 113. *2* | 132. *3* | 151. *1* | |
| 19. *1* | 38. *1* | 57. *3* | 76. *1* | 95. *1* | 114. *2* | 133. *1* | 152. *4* | |